C000181515

The Compleat Distiller

Benj. Ormond Perry: Surgeon

Bastard S[t] Christophers

April 8th 1748

Benjamin Ormond

Perry Surgeon

55,97

Ben Ormond THE Poney

Compleat Distiller:

Malimba OR THE Africa

Whole ART 1742

OF

DISTILLATION

Practically Stated,

And Adorned with all the New Modes of WORKING now in Use.

In which is Contained,

The Way of making Spirits, Aquavitæ, Artificial Brandy, and their Application to Simple and Compound Waters in the exact *Pondus* of the Greater and Lesser Composition; as also many Curious and Profitable Truths for the exalting of Liquors, being the Epitomy and Marrow of the whole Art; supplying all that is omitted in the *London Distiller*, *French Baker*, &c. Experience being the true Polisher hereof.

To which is Added,

Pharmacopœia Spagyrica nova: Or an Helmontian Course; being a Description of the Philosophical *Sal-Armoniack*, *Volatile Salt* of *Tartar*, and *Circulatum Minus*, &c. Together with their Use and Office in Preparing *Powers*, *Arcanums*, *Magisteries*, and *Quintessences*, the Dose and Vertues being Annexed.

The *Second Edition*, with Alterations and Additions.

Illustrated with Copper Sculptures.

By *W. Y-Worth*, Medicinæ Professor in Doctrinis Spagyricis & per Ignem Philosophus.

London, Printed for J. Taylor, at the *Ship* in St. *Paul*'s Church-Yard. MDCCV.

THE

Epistle to the READER.

Courteous Reader,

THE *End and Intention of our Writing and Compiling these Sheets, is to bring the* Art *of* Distillation *into one compleat and entire Volume, containing all the necessaries thereunto belonging: For hitherto this hath been but short and defectively performed, for it hath had the mishap, as many other excellent Arts have had,* &c. *To be Treated of by such, as have not practically known the same; or else by those, who have on purpose concealed that, which in reality ought to have been discovered; so that the Authors hitherto extant are either filled with needless Prescriptions, confused Workings, long and tedious Prolixity of Words and Circumlocutions, as we may say, going about the Wood, or else have concealed the* Ariadnean *thread, which should lead directly to the Practick, and so are only useful to those, who have served seven Years Apprentiship to the imploy, then knowing what to choose and what to refuse, and being able to pick the Rose from among Thorns without pricking themselves; for what a chargable and confused piece of work should we have, were we to provide our selves with all those Vessels and Instruments described by* Baker, *for the making* Waters, Aqua vitæ, *and* Burning Spirits, *and to separate them from the Flegm; which, when done, would neither answer the end nor countervail the charge; for 'tis well known to all ingenious Men, how difficult a thing it was to prepare a Spirit, which would fire Gun-powder, or be so purely Ætherial as to vanish in the Sun, 'till the use of Salt was known, by whose help we are able to perform it in large quantities, even in our common Stills with their Refrigeratory; And the most exact way that we ever saw is to work with Salts in a large Copper Body with its Alembick and Refrigeratory in* Baln. *For with a lent heat you will have your Spirit perfectly deflegm'd, which for curiosity sake, you may repeat a second time, and then will it far excel any of those made by the difficult Inventions before mentioned; and therefore why should we go to so much charge and trouble, when it may be performed with so much facility and ease: And again,*

gain, he is filled with abundance of Chymical Preparations, which have not the least adherence to the making of Spirits; and so the mind of the Reader is diverted from that, which only should be of Service to him; nay, this is so apt to fill their heads with fancies, that they rest unsatisfied 'till brought to Tryals, which either considerably exhaust their Substance, or else take them from their Business, nay, sometimes wholy incapacitates them for the same; therefore shall we pass by him; and come to consider that of French.

Dr. French *indeed was a Man of Ingenuity, as his Work plainly shows, seeing many curious things are therein contained, yet can we not wholly clear him from some of these Defects.*

And as for the London Distiller, *tho' his Prescriptions, there laid down are proper, yet is he defective, both in the exact* Modus *of working, the ordering of the* Wash *and* Backs *for a quick Fermentation, and upon a defect in their working to bring them kindly forward again; as also in the great Business of Rectification, concerning which there is so great a noise about the*

Town;

Town; and indeed not without good reason, seeing too too many are deficient in so advantageous a Secret as this is; yet is both he and French *so scarce, that one of them is hardly to be gotten; and then again on the other hand, what we have formerly written, in order to have supplied these Defects, was in such general Terms and so short, as that of it self it was not sufficient to make any one prompt-perficient in the Art.*

Therefore we being desired by several Ingenious Persons to communicate our Experience to the World, and so to supply the defects before mentioned, as much as in us lay, have upon a mature Consideration thereunto condescended, with this Resolution, that we would do it so as to capacitate any one, tho' of a mean Genius, *and never brought up to the Art, in a little time by Study and Practice to be a compleat Master in the same, without having recourse to any other Author; for which end we have comprised it into a Pocket-Volume, that so it might be the more portable, and by consequence ready for their Perusal.*

Now that you may the better conceive what is therein contained, we shall in brief pro-

proceed, as follows; In the first place, we have described the manner of Working in general with all the necessary Utensils thereunto belonging, and then in a more particular way have shewed various and profitable ways of making Low-wines *from any of the six Materials; some by Decoction, and others without, giving you our Opinion which we best approve of, we have indeed here laid down such Rules in the ways of Brewing and Ordering the Wash, as also in the bringing it into* Low-wines, *as that there is no Material in Nature that will yield a Vinous Spirit, but what may be wrought by some or other of them; and being thus far brought, the time of their lying for their bettering is signified, together with the way of bringing them into* Proof-goods; *And then,*

In the Second we have shown the exact way of Rectification, by and through such Mediums, *as that they are brought into most excellent* Stuff, *and if the use of* Tartar *and* Sulphur *whether common or that of* Mars *and* Venus, *joyned with the sweet Salt were known, certainly sweet and pleasant Spirits might be brought forth; but more especially by the help of our* Sal Panaristos

ristos *might* English *goods be so ordered as that in Tast and Smell they might be little inferior to those of* Gallia, *and equal in Vertue to the* English *Constitutions; because of their Climatary Affinity, concerning which, we have not only given you our own Experience, but also the Authority of the famous* Radolphus Glauber; *which being so prepared we have likewise shown their various uses in making* Cordial-Waters *and* Spirits.

In the Third, we have shown all the Necessary *and Useful Compositions in the Art, according to the greater and lesser* Pondus; *to which we have added many rare ones of our own, togethet with an* Usque-baugh-Royal, *never Published before, and also the way of Dulcifying and Perfuming these Wares or Liquors, so that they may be the most Commodious for Sale.*

In the Second Part we have laid down the true and Genuine way of making Powers *by three noble* Menstruums, sc. *a* Purified Circulatum Minus, *the* Volatile Salt *of* Tartar, *and* Sal Panaristos, *together with their Vertues, Use and Dose, for the Benefit of such, as languish under the burthen*

then of Refractory Diseases, and can find no Relief from the common Prescriptions; for we have through much Expence and Labour by the Providence of God thereunto attained, and by more than Ten Years Experience, know their admirable Vertues to be such, as to relieve, when past the hopes of other means; therefore we thought we could not better befriend the World, especially the ingenious Lovers of Art, than freely to communicate their Composition, that so they might the better judge of their Nature and Property; and altho' we have not attributed so many Vertues thereunto, as others have done to more Inferiour Powers, *yet this hath been on purpose omitted for two Reasons: The first, because we hate fruitless Repetitions, or to speak more of the Vertues and Use of Things, than we know they will really perform; for we would rather that a Medicine should Cure Ten Diseases, when we speak but of five, than to speak of* Forty, *when 'twill very rarely Cure One; and especially in these, seeing their Administration is general and safe without the least difficulty: The other is, because we have looked upon it as a grand Error too often committed by our* New Compiler, *to attribute that to one sleight or common* **Pre-***paration, which can but in due right be a-scribed to the highest* Specifick *or* Arcanum, *nay, even to the* Universal *it self; there-fore, tho' we know that ours are far superior, yet were we resolved therein to be very cau-tious, least others should suppose us guilty of the like default.*

Now, what we have further to say, is, that we have great reason to bless the Lord our God, who of his infinite Mercy hath given us Wisdom and Knowledge of the things of Nature, not only in their Original *Form and Texture, but also in their true Preparati-on and Vertue, whereby we are enabled to demonstrate that, which we doubt not will uphold our Writings in a greater splendor than now set forth; to the dishonour of such, as are ambitious of that which really does be-long to others; but seeing ours is no Foster-child, but a true birth brought forth by diffi-cult Travel, we are bound to defend it from the Carps of such* Momes, *and the more especially seeing we have daily Confirmati-ons, from most parts of the Kingdom, of its kind acceptance, by, and among, the Ingeni-ous, Laborious and Honest-hearted, which*

lays

lays a further Obligation on us to be yet as serviceable to such as in us lies, in the resolution of which we subscribe our selves their sincere Friend in all things agreeable to the entire Law of Innocency.

From my House, the *Blew Ball* and *Star* at the corner of *King street* in upper *Morefields, London*,

W. Y-Worth, *Geboortigh tot* Shipham, & *Burger van* Rotterdam.

THE

CONTENTS,

Or Chief HEADS of the first Part, of the Compleat Distiller.

Of

The CONTENTS.

 making

Aqua

The CONTENTS.

The CONTENTS.

The

The CONTENTS *of the Second Part*, viz. **Pharmacopæia Spagyrica.**

Pote-

The CONTENTS.

Pote-

Aurum

A De

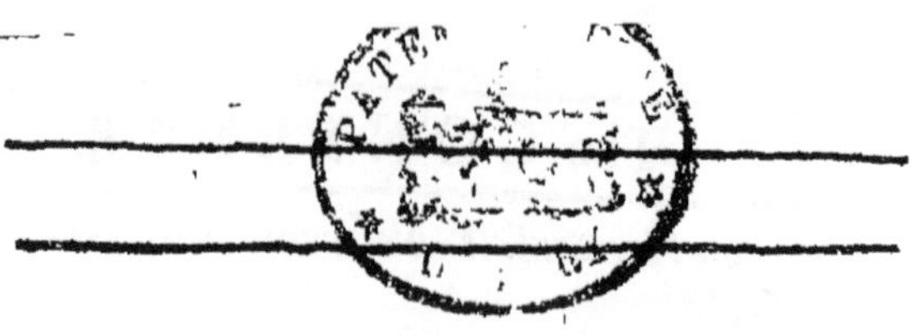

ADVERTISEMENT.

MY Father has communicated to me these well known and deservedly Famous Medicines, for their approved Vertues, and general benefit in Curing Diseases, *viz. Spiritus Mundus*, *Essentia Munda*, *Spiritus Sedativus*, or *Elixir Proprietatis Helmontii*, *Essentia Stomatica*, *Species Mineralis*, *Arcanum Minerale*, *Species Antipileptic*, and *Species Lithontriptic*, &c. In their highest Exaltation of Vertue they can be brought to, being prepared by an Universal *Medium*, and advanced by a Mineral *Pacative* Sulphur, yet their Fragrancy dignified; Medicines eminently known and approved of, for many Years, by thousands, for the Cure of Agues, Fevers, *Pleurisies*, Measles, Small pox, Swine-pox, Surfeits, *&c.* And for all *Pestilential* Diseases are superlative Specificks, also in the Gripes, Cholick, Quinsey, and other acute Diseases: And for Cronick and Refractory ones you have my *Pillula Herculeana*, which cures all those Taints that are received in the Schools of *Venus*, even when spoiled by others, without Salivation or hindrance of Business, with a very few Doses, and at little Charge: 'Tis also excellent against Itch, Scab, and Leprosie, and all grand Corruptions of the Blood, Ulcers, Festula's, and *Noli me Tangere's*. As to Lunatick Persons, or such as are afflicted with Melancholly Madness, or those Raving, in consideration of the

the chargable, tedious and prolix Methods that are now used by so many Upstarts, and yet so little advantage to the Patients, that they are kept year after year, we think convenient to inform the Friends of such, that we have a more certain and established Method for the Cure of all that are Curable, which is exhibited after a Christian way, without Tyranny or cruel Scourging, being radical Specificks for that Disease, which restore to Sense and pristine Vigour.

All which Medicines are faithfully prepared by **Theophrastus P-Worth**, and may be had at reasonable Rates, either by Wholesale or Retail, at the *Blew-ball and Star*, the corner House of *King-street* in upper *Morefields*, *London*.

At which place may be also had his Famous *Spiritus Odontugiasus*, which whitens black and yellow Teeth, in few Minutes, and cures the Scurvy in the Mouth, and Defects of the Gums, *&c.*

Now, whereas, my Father appearing in Print, has occasion'd great Recourse of Letters, these are to Advertise, that for the future they direct them to me at the place abovesaid, which (the Postage being paid) shall be faithfully Communicated to my Father; otherwise not received: And if an Answer is expected, they are desired to subscribe their Names and Place of Habitation, because he has been so often Imposed on by several who have desired to be satisfied in many curious Inquiries, *&c.* Who yet have refused the Candour of Communicating,

municating their Name, &c. Or shewing the Reason why they should be Answer'd.

ERRATA.

PAge 43. *Line* 6. for knew, *Read* new, *p*. 70. *l*. 14. for Ugar, *r*. Sugar. *p*. 90. *l*. 6. for Balm, *r*. Bawm. *p*. 110. *l*. 2. for aucrified, *r*. aurified. *p*. 124. for Trepoile, *r*. Trefoil. *p*. 176. *l*. 10. for Chilbane, *r*. Bane. *p*. 180. *l*. 10. for Pledge, *r*. Pledget. *p*. 198. *l*. 27. for as, *r*. us. *p*. 225. for ture, *r*. true. *p*. 227. *l*. 19. for Ensentificated, *r*. Essentificated. *p*. 235. *l*. 29. for Dustan, *r*. Dunstan. *p*. 236. *l*. 2. for it, *r*. in. *l*. 17. adding. *r*. according. *p*. 238. *l*. 13. for Party, *r*. Purity. *p*. 253. *l*. *ult*. for Poable, *r*. Potable. *p*. 267. *l*. 5. Alagistrale, *r*. Magistrale.

THE

THE Compleat Distiller.

4.7.18.

CHAP. I.

In which we Treat of the Art of Distillation in general, together with the Utensils thereunto belonging.

FIRST, We think it convenient to define the word *Distillation*, and then to shew the use thereof; the word Distillation imports no more than *a dropping down by little and little*; but the use and end thereof, is in the first place to Extract the Spirituality from bodies, when macerated or open'd by Fermentation; so that we may truly say this Art is for changing of gross and thick bodies into a thin and Spiritual Nature, by which Action the pure *Effluvia* are separated from the more terrene, Fætid, and impure *Faces*; and that only by the help of heat; they being thereby resolved into a Vapour, are elevated to the Helm, where they are in part condensed by the cold, which is fully accomplished, as they run out of the Beck into the Worm, through the Refrigerating Tub, and so become clear and lucid: This is the end of Distillation in general, but in particular, 'tis to be considered in a threefold respect, *sc. Distillation, Rectification*, and *Extraction*; **Distillation** *is a converting of Bodies* (as before defined) *into Water, Oyl and Spirit*; **Rectification** *is a reiterated Elevation, by which the before mentioned are separated from their more hidden and internal Impurities; and the Spiritual, Essential humidity, from the more Phlegmatick and Aqueous*: *And* **Extraction** *is by the help of some pure Spirit to draw forth that virtue out of bodies, which otherwise would not so easily admit of Maceration, or of being so overcome, as to be brought into Spirituallity*: Now in bodies very compact, this is best performed by *Cohobation*, which is a returning the Liquor upon the Body whence Extracted, and Distilling it off again; which must so often be repeated as till you've obtained the desired Virtues; these being sufficient to accomplish all that is to be expected from a *Distiller*, and indeed to make the Art compleat, and the Discourse thereof full, seeing we intend not to speak of any thing but what is pertinent thereunto, we shall refer those who desire to know the Nature of other Operations, to our *Chymicus Rationalis*, where they are fully and amply handled, and so passing by the use and Definition of this Art, we shall now come to the Practick.

In which we find that it requires a great many Conveniences, as a fit Work-house, proper Stills, Coppers, Backs, Instruments and Materials, all which, to be rightly managed, require several hands, if any considerable draught

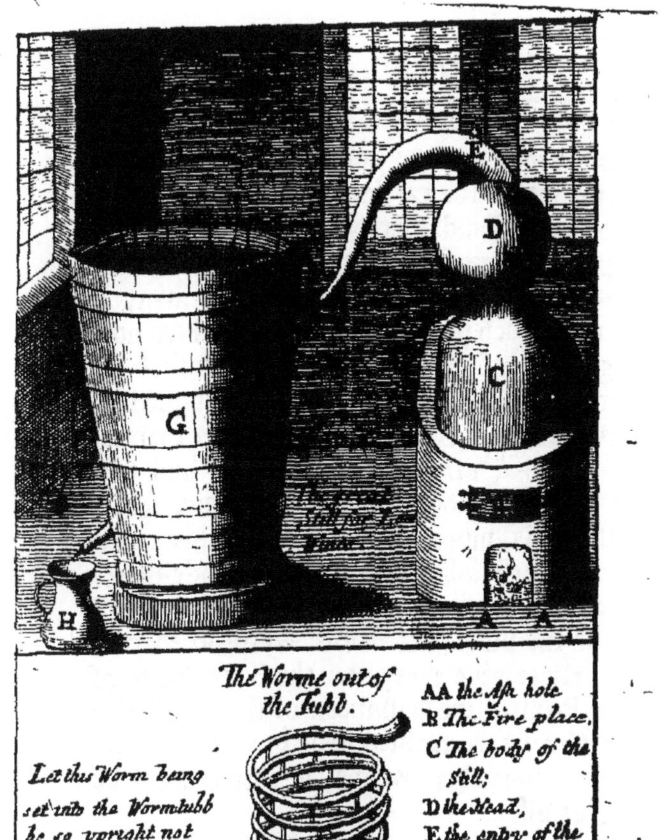

The Worme out of the Tubb.

Let this Worm being set into the Wormtubb be so upright not inclining to the right or left hand, but so ye water being put in it may run out to a drop.

AA *the Ash hole*
B *The Fire place.*
C *The body of the Still;*
D *the Head,*
E *the entry of the Crane neck:*
F *the joyning of ye nose thereof to the Worme,*
G *the Worme tubb,*
H *the Can;*

Place this Figure before Chap: I in page. 11.

draught of Goods is intended to be made, so from hence we may conclude that this Art is not rightly to be carried on without a considerable large Fund, but when so managed 'twill repay the Owner, or Master with considerable Interest; which is the reason that many of them get such plentiful Estates, at which none ought to grudge, seeing 'tis got with such just gain, and that the Golden Cap is obtained by hard Labour: And besides, there's a Proverb in *England*, *win Gold and wear it*; and why therefore may not these enjoy the same, seeing nothing is more laborious than this Art, when rightly followed; and what they thereby obtain, we may, as it were, say, is got out of the Fire: But before we proceed particularly to give every one the Knowledge of these Profits, we shall speak of the necessaries whereby we are enabled to go to work, otherwise without them we may be sure there'll be none at all.

First, As to the Work-house, we best esteem it when something spacious, at least 16, 18, or 20 Foot in breadth; and 24, 26, 28, or 30, in length; especially, where you design to work considerable quantities. The manner of Erecting the Carcase with the proportionable height, and way of covering it, we shall leave to the Ingenuity of the Work-man, to whom it belongs, and give you our Opinion of the Accomplishment of what is required in it: Thus, at the utmost end we advise that a Copper be set up, after the manner of the *Brewers*; except you design to prepare your Liquor in your large Still, which will be somewhat troublesome, and indeed a great hinderance to business, if you intend to work it off twice a day, as usually is done: Now by your Copper you must have your Mashing Tub, to mash in; and under that large Receivers, and over upon the Rafters you may have a Cooler; and again under the Coolers large Backs, one for the stronger Wort, the other for the smaller; and so order'd, as that it may run into either; now from these large Backs, you must convey Leaden Pipes unto receiving Backs for Stores, and from your store ones to the Wash-backs, which ought always to be placed opposite to your great Stills, for the more ready filling of them; now this conveyance is very convenient, from Back to Back; for by this means you may always be supplied with Wash; and especially if you command it by the turning of a Cock, otherwise you must make use of a strong Cork with a String above it, that so you may pluck it out when you please. Now these Backs, as they are set into the Earth, must be well daubed about with temper'd Clay, or put in a thin Bed thereof; for this is said to preserve them tight and warm: These must have Covers above with a Leaf to fold up upon occasion; and upon a defect of Backs, you may make use of large Oyl Fats, so order'd; you must have a Brass or Wooden Pump to put into the Backs, and so with a Spout fastned with a Broom therein, to keep the Wash from running over, and the other

end

end on the Still you would fill, you may at any time eaſily perform it; your Spout being moveable from Still to Still.

In hanging your Stills you muſt obſerve, to place them on the ſame ſide that your Copper is on, that ſo your Backs may be the better ranged together without Confuſion; let them be as near the end as they'll poſſibly ſtand; and let two ſtand together, that ſo one Flew may ſerve for the conveyance of both their Smoaks; and in the firſt place you muſt obſerve to place them ſo, as that the lower end of the Worm may be 14 Inches from the Ground, that ſo a Can may freely be placed under, and taken away when full: 'tis better an Inch too high than a quarter of one too low; and for proportioning your Still to any height, you muſt let in your Aſh-hole into the ground; which in length and breadth muſt be proportionable to that of the Still; for one of ſix Barrels ten or twelve Inches in breadth is ſufficient; and for one of eight or ten Barrels, it muſt be twelve or fourteen at the leaſt; the which are two very good Sizes; the length muſt be proportioned according to the Grate and Door, ſomewhat ſloping for the more eaſie commanding the Aſhes. And having proceeded thus far, you muſt obſerve not to make the fire place too broad: your Grate muſt be made of thick heavy Bars, exactly cut, of an even length, the ends ſomewhat flatted upon flat Bars, and broad, flat Bars muſt lie even with their upper edges, that ſo the Shovel, Slice or Rake may not jam in them, although they lie loose, to be taken in or out upon occasion as any of them melt off: The broad flat Bars must be continued tight one to another, even to the mouth of the Door; and the Door must be of Iron, as the Brewers Coppers are; let your mouth and fire place be built all of broad Tiles, for these better bear the fury of the Fire than Bricks: And when your Fire place is of its proper height, and at one end a convenient sloping hole left for the Fire to play up in, let your Still be placed upon the Brick-work, in such a way as that it may have a Current for the Liquor to run out of the Cock; and upon tryal let it be closely work'd up to the bottom, that so the Fire may only play at the Flew; and observe to place your Cocks through the Wall, that so the Liquor or Wash may run out into the proper receiving Backs, without annoying the Still-house. Let there be a Wheel-vent made to receive the Smoak and Flame, at least five, six, seven, or eight Inches, as your Still is in bigness, which taking the Fire throws it round the Still, and brings it into the great Flew or Chimney; 'tis generally ordered, that the Wheel-vent should go with the Sun; but if you hang two Stills together, which is the right way, then let the one Vent go to the right and the other to the left, that so both may the easier meet in the great Flew; or you may continue their division to what height you please by a Brick on the edge between them. The Wall of your Stills must go with an exact round, and be carried up only the

thick-

thickness of a Brick. Between the Angle of the two rounds, let flat Bars be fastned two or three like a Ladder, that so you may go up to see, when the Still is full; as also to cleanse it upon occasion. When your Work is carried up as high as the upper Nails in the Still, then cover your Vent, by carrying on your Work sloping 'till you come to the narrow place of the Still; let the edge of your Work be round, that so, if any Liquor fall on the Slope, it may the easier drop away; your work above being well secured all round with plain Tiles and a good bed of Mortar, then you must cover your Still all round with a course Canvass, or Hop-Sack, in order to keep the Walls from cracking, and the Fire tighter or more closely in; which must also be exactly Plaistered and White-limed over: Your Still being thus hung and finished, we shall now come to consider the placing of the Worm-Tub.

Now in this you must observe to set it on a Wall made of Brick with some Timber in it, which must be covered with a round board like the Curb of a Well, the better to keep it from sinking, the Board must be the exact Compass of the Bottom of the Tub, but the Wall something less, that so a Can may the better stand before it: And here you must observe these Rules, **First**, *That the upper end of your Worm stand so that the Beck or Nose of the Head may easily go into the same without the least Obstruction, and shut in so close, as easily to be luted*: **Secondly**, *That your Worm-tub must stand*

 upright

upright, leaning neither one way nor another; otherwiſe the Liquor will hang in the Worm: **Thirdly,** *To try whether the Worm be upright, that you may put a Pint or a Quart of Water in the ſame, and if it comes all out of the lower end, then may you aſſure your ſelf 'tis true;* which being regarded you can't miſs of ſetting your Tub a-right.

Moreover, we approve beſt of thoſe Helms, which have a large Pewter Crane Neck, proceeding from the upper Center of the Head into the Worm, for two Reaſons; the one is becauſe the Spirits come ſweeter through this ſort than that of the Copper; the other is, that if the Waſh ſhould riſe into the Head, yet will it not ſo readily come over to foul the Worm. Laſtly, you muſt have two or three Loops or Ears in the upper part of your Head to tye a Rope, that ſo by the help of a Pully you may the eaſier lift off the ſame: This Still head, and Worm-tub are exactly deſcribed in Fig.

Thus having ſhown you the manner of hanging the Still, ſetting the Worm-tub, &c. and alſo given demonſtration thereof to your Eye, in the Figure; we ſhall now come to ſhew the way of preparing things fit to be therein Diſtilled; as alſo the manner of working the ſame.

Now the *Baſis* or Grounds for Diſtillation may be comprehended under theſe ſix Heads: **Firſt,** *Ale, and Liquors brewed and prepared from Malt, by any way of extraction or drawing forth whatſoever.* **Secondly,** *All things, that*

are

are to be Brewed and Diſtilled from Molaſſes Sugar and Honey, either with or without Tilts: **Thirdly**, *All thoſe, which are or may be made from Fruits, Berries and Flowers of the* Engliſh *growth, as, Cyder, Perry, and Artificial Wines:* **Fourthly**, *Thoſe of Foreign Fruits, as, Raiſings, Figs, Prunes, Tamarinds, or others, that either may by Art be Brewed, or will give a Spirit by Fermentation:* **Fifthly**, *All kind of Foreign Wines, and their Lees:* **Sixthly**, *All kind of Herbs whatſoever, either with or without Addition.*

Theſe being ſufficient to demonſtrate all that can be ſaid in the Art, are laid down, to the end, that you may the better conceive of, and comprehend, what is to be ſpoken thereof, in the particular ways of Working: We ſhall now begin with the firſt Head, that of Malt.

In which there are various ways of working, one Brewing it into ſound Ale and Beer, which is the beſt, and letting it come to Age and Strength before Diſtilled; others Brewing it without any Boyling or Hops, bringing the three Liquors together into their Waſh-backs, and ſo Ferment and Diſtil; others Ferment Malted Wheat and Malt, and ſo Diſtil; and others are for Protuberating and burſting Corn by boyling of it, and then Fermenting and Diſtilling it; all which ſhall be treated of apart. And firſt of Brewing ſound Beer, becauſe from thence the beſt and trueſt *Aqua Vitæ*'s are made.

As

As to Brewing we have given you our opinion in our *Cerevisiarii Comes*, which in short is, that by Decoction the destructive *Gass* must be taken out of the Water, and then to be cool'd in, which is, that some of it must be cold, and as much put on the Malt as will serve for mixtion and commixtion; and then pouring on as much warm Liquor as you intend to make use of in that Mashing; then rowing up well, and letting it stand its due time, to draw it into the Receivers, and so to proceed, as directed in the before-cited Book; only you are to observe, that if it should not be fully rich of the Malt, to Distil it as soon as 'tis well wrought, for fear it should flat, and so great part of the Spirit should be lost; but if it be very Strong and well Brewed, you may keep it to what Age you please, before you Distil it. The way to Distil it will be shown hereafter.

The second is the general way made use of by all the *Distillers*; the way whereof though laid down in the precited Book, shall be here again repeated, because this may come into the hands of those, which that may not, and because we design in this to make the Art compleat and entire. First, you are to heat your Water a little above Blood warm, *i. e.* between Blood-warm and scalding hot, but observe, that you take it before it breaks, which they call Pinch O' my Nail; for, they say, *that if you boyl your Liquor you make it hard, and so 'twill not take out the Virtue of your Malt*, but we know to the contrary, for if the Liquor

quor is so boyled, as that only the *Gass* may evaporate, little or no Consumption being made, it is by that means made more mellow, and will extract more virtue out of the Malt, if in a good temper put thereto, and then the Malt being in a Mash-tub, add so much Liquor to it as is just sufficient to wet it, and this is called *Mashing*; then row or stir it up very well with two or three pair of Hands, stiffly for half an hour together, till 'tis all mixed in every part; then add in what quantity of Liquor you think fit; but the stiffer you Mash, the better it is; then strow it all over with a little fresh Malt, and let it stand an hour and a quarter, or thereabouts; then let it off into its Receivers, and Mash again with fresh Liquor, and let it stand about an hour, rowing it up, as before said; so a third time: And some will Mash a fourth time, which then must not stand above half an hour: But we say that three times are sufficient; the fourth being so poor and very small indeed, that 'tis fitter for Small-beer for very poor People, than for a Distillation; unless 'tis used instead of Liquor for other Mashings on fresh Malt. Now some very Ingenious Persons Boyl their Liquor and Cool it, the which we well approve of.

Now every Wort that comes is pump'd up out of the under Back into the Cooler, there to Cool; and then from the Cooler into the Wash-backs, there to remain 'till all the three Worts come together. By the way observe, that you neither Hop nor Boyl, as for Beer; now

now when they are down in the Backs, and in a proper coolness and fit to be set; then add good Yeast enough to work it very well, as for Ale; and as the Yeast rises up beat it down again, and keep the same all in; and let it work three, four, or five days, according to the Season of the Year, Temperament of your Back, when set, and Judgment of the Distiller.

If a Back be set either too cold or too hot, 'tis thus holpen, by adding either hot or cold Liquors, to bring it unto a good Temperature; in the Winter time, in extream cold weather when it flats and goes backward, and will come to no good Head; you may again promote it's Fermentation by adding some of those things prescribed in that of *Molasses*: Now if you can exactly know the time of the Wash's being come, then you may take off your thick Yeast, to set other Backs with: But if not, then must you take with you these signs, *sc.* the working it self down flat, and then the thick Yeast sinking to the bottom, that so what lies on the top will be but a kind of an Hoary or Yeasty Head: You must observe that your Wash be neither sowre nor sweet, but in a *Medium* between both; for't will then be most profitable for Distillation: but some say, that being taken in its highest Curle, before it begin to flat, and the Yeast and all Stilled, it gives the most Spirit; the way whereof will be also hereafter shown.

The third we call the *Dutch way*, because mostly used in *Holland* and *Germany*, which is, is, the Fermenting of the Corn; which to do, you muſt proceed thus: Take freſh ground Malt, made of Wheat, Barley, or Buck Wheat, *&c.* and put it into the Oyl Tubs before deſcribed, pouring thereon as much cold Water as will ſerve for mixtion and commixtion, and then alſo pouring as much warm Water, as will ſuffice for making the mixture moiſt and thin, alſo warm, for it muſt be neither hot nor cold, but in the *Medium* between both; which being done, and well rowed up, mix therewith ſome new Barm, and cover it with its Cover and Cloth very warm; which being expoſed to the Heat will in a ſhort ſpace begin to Ferment; therefore you are not to fill your Veſſels above three quarters full; this you muſt leave until Fermented, and the mixture deſcends, which for the moſt part will be on the third or fourth day; and then is it ready for Diſtillation; but 'tis generally experienced by thoſe which are not uſed to this way, that the Malt, being put into the Still Cakes and burns to the bottom, to the deſtruction both of the ſame, and *Low-wines*, which come off with a burnt taſte; which to prevent, there are two ways; the one is to preſs forth the Liquor from the Grains, and to Diſtil the ſame; the other is by our new Invention, which will be ſhown hereafter; for we ſaw that all our Experiments made in a boyling Bath did not in the leaſt burn; but that all the *Low-wines* came off very ſweet and luſcious in taſte, and pleaſant in ſmell.

The

The Fourth and Laſt, is the *Glauberian* way, which is thus: Firſt, you muſt after this manner prepare your Corn, whether Barley, Rie, Oats, or Wheat; *&c.* ſteep it in ſweet Water for ſome days, then place it, that it may ſprout after the ſame manner as Corn is Malted for the making of Beer; turn it well for a certain time, leſt it be corrupted by too much heat; then when it is well ſprouted, ſpread it abroad, that it may preſently cool, and 'twill never ſowre.

But if you would uſe it preſently, then take as much of it as your Diſtillation will require, and in a Kettle full of Water, boyl it ſo long, till the Grains are broken, then pour it into a Wooden Veſſel, and when it is luke-warm, add to it the freſh Dregs or Grounds of Beer, and let it Ferment; when it has fermented enough, which is uſually at the end of two or three days, then *Brandy-wine* is made in a common Still, by Diſtillation from that Corn; what remains in the Still will ſerve to feed Oxen, Cows, Hogs, or other Cattle.

But the *Brandy-wine* which proceeds from thence muſt be rectified, as the way is; and by this means 'tis render'd more ſweet and grateful to the Reliſh, than any other *Brandy* made of Corn: the Reaſon is this, That all Bread-Corn, of which *Brandy-wine* ought to be prepared, if it be put to Ferment preſently after ſoftning, is neceſſarily in the Still, by boiling, reduced into a Pap, and ſo being corrupted by aduſtion produces a ſtinking *Brandy-wine*.

But

But this protuberated and burst Corn cannot be burnt, and therefore makes good *Brandy*.

Now 'tis observable that that *Brandy* made from Wheat-Corn, is the most near of any other from any Grain whatsoever, to that of *Gallia*, and gives good quantity of Spirits: So doth Rie and Buck-wheat, being Protuberated. and yields very large quantities of Spirits, if distilled according to the new way of our Patentees in Tubs, and as *Glauber* has described; and you may see the manner of it at Mr. *Hollands*, below *Limos-bridge*; which way I very much approve of for the Distilling of whole and protuberated Grain.

Let thus much at present suffice concerning Corn, because the distinct rules of bringing it into *Low-wines*, *Proof Spirits*, and *Rectified Goods*, will be laid down in their proper Places; we shall therefore now proceed to the second Head; *sc. Molasses*, *Sugar* and *Honey*.

As to *Molasses*, you need to do no more, than down with it into the Backs (seeing for promise sake we must open so many Truths) and add thereto three or four times its weight of Liquor, prepared as in the second Head; *i. e.* to every Hundred of *Molasses* thirty six, forty, or forty six Gallons of Liquor, according as you will have it small or rich of the *Molasses*; for you must observe, that the stronger it is, the longer 'twill be before it comes to Fermentation; and this, if it be not well Fermented, will yield but poorly, *i. e.* very little quantity of Spirits, therefore is it abun-

abundantly nicer to be wrought than that of Malt; and especially in these cold Climates; for you must observe to set your Back at once in a good temper; being not so well to be holpen by hot or cold Liquors, as that of Corn; and you must have good store of Yeast, or Ferment to Head it well at once, or else it will not come on; but if you use Wash instead of Water and Tilts, the Grounds of very strong Beer, will help its Fermentation on so, that abundantly less Yeast will serve; and you must observe, that it stands, especially in the Winter time, in a very warm Place; and if in the second day it should not begin to come well on, the which it will not, if set either too hot or too cold; then you must have ready by you a Pot of very strong Mustard, with a Horse-raddish and good Onion, and the value of an Egg, or two of these must be cast in; you may dip the Onion and Horse-Raddish in the Mustard; and this will highly promote its Fermentation; especially if you add a Ball of Whiting; Tartar or Argal is not to be despised in the Doctrine of Fermentation; for 'twill give a secret and sure internal one, yet when a Back is in too high a Foam, 'twill kindly flat it: In all this you must observe, that Experience must be your chief guide; for tho' we discover true things, yet several accidents may occur, wherein this Mistress may and will be your best help: For you must know that when it is truly Fermented, you must take it in the right Nick, neither too high nor too flat, neither to sweet

nor

nor too sowre; for by any extream, you may lose of your quantity of Spirit, as well as by the want of due Fermentation; therefore if a Back of *Molasses* have not yielded you Spirit enough, let it cool, fit to set again, and then add in a few Gallons of fresh Treacle, stir them well together, and Ferment with Ale Yeast and a Ball of Whiting, as before, and so draw a second time Ingenious Reader! make not strange of this working over of *Molasses* a second time, seeing it hath been often done; and we are credibly informed by a Person of Ingenuity, that in *Barbados* and those Islands where the Sugar Canes are in large quantity, *they take the* Molasses, *foul* Sugar, *and their* Canes, *and Ferment them together with remains of the former Distillation, and upon a defect of Fermentation they cast in some Wood-Ashes newly made, together with some live Coals. He farther said, that when it is almost brought to its height in Fermentation, they add five Gallons more of* Molasses, *and then stir and Ferment, as before, and then again five Gallons, always keeping it in Fermentation, and with other reiterate additions proceed until it is very rich of the* Molasses: But if so, then are they in this Case beholding to their Climate for the Heat, which helps on their Fermentation; for here that would not be performed under a long and tedious time, therefore we shall omit it; but as for the using their remains we much credit, because it carries with it so strong an Hogo; the way of bringing it into *Low-wines, Proof Goods, and Rectified Spirits* will be shown in its proper place.

Honey must be mixed with four, five, six, seven, or eight parts of warm Water, and dissolved; and then to the Solution you must add Ferment, as was spoken concerning Malt, which afterwards must be left covered in some heat for to be Fermented; being fit for Distillation when it comes to wax hot. Now know that too great a quantity of Honey makes a very slow Fermentation, *viz.* of some Weeks or Months; wherefore for acceleration sake we advise, that a greater quantity of Water be added, although otherwise it yields plenty of Spirits, but ungrateful; which therefore we would have no body to Distil, as being unprofitable, unless any one know how to take away the ungratefulness thereof; which will be more largely shown in the Chapter of Rectification: *Low-wines, Proof Goods* and *Rectified Spirits*, may be made from those *Meads* described in our *Britannean Magazine* of *Wine*; and most excellent and flavorous Spirits they are indeed: Moreover as to what concerns Sugar, it may be performed by what is laid down of *Molasses* and *Honey*, and therefore being needless to repeat it, we shall pass on to another Head.

Now as to Cyder, Perry, and Artificial Wines, together with such Liquors as may be made from *English* growths, according to the general way commonly known, as also that already prescribed in our *Britannean Magazine*, they being well Fermented, and by Age come to be ripe and fine, there is no difficulty to obtain there from a generous Spirit. Note, that

that Cyders yield but little quantity of Spirit, let them be made never so fine by age; therefore 'tis requisite that you again open them, and bring them to a fresh Ferment, and then they will yield plentifully; also when they are declining, prick'd, ropy or flat, it is requisite that they be again helped into a Fermentative State, by such additions as will measurably revive them; sometimes Whites of Eggs and Flour will do it; or some *Alkalisated Calx*; and if not, then must you proceed to your common way, and Ferment, by which and warmth new Cyder may be so brought as in five, six, or seven days it will be fit to be Distilled; and so of the rest. Now among many *fine Goods*, excellent *Stuff* may be made from sound Fruits, especially Cyder; that so with small additions good *Brandies* may be made; therefore why should we contemn the perfect Knowledge of *Molasses* and *Cider-Spirits*, seeing by a little Industry great things may thereby be performed: But what is here said being sufficient for all kind of Fruits, seeing the Doctrine of Fermentation is elsewhere more largely laid down; passing this by, we shall come to the fourth Head.

Raisings, Figs and other Foreign Fruits, may either be stamped in a great Stone Mortar, or put down whole into your Backs, adding warm Liquor to them, as in the second Head of Corn, and as the Back is fit to be set, add thereunto your common Ferment, and with a due heat they will kindly come forward, and as the Fruit arises at the Top, you may beat them down again; but if they work not kindly in the ſecond or third day, then you may add in a Ball of Whiting, or a ſmall Portion of *Calx Viva* or *Argal*, not forgeting the helps before mentioned. We alſo have ſeen excellent effects from *Chryſtals* of *Tartar*: For thus we have made moſt excellent Wines, according as is touched at in our *Britannean Magazine*. Now as ſoon as they are fully Fermented, which will ſometimes be a Day ſooner than at other times, you may Diſtil them, their Juice being either preſt out, or the Fruit put into the Still, as we in our Tryals have ſometimes done; but then we have obſerved often to take off the Head, and ſtir them, till ready to boyl, for fear they ſhould Cake: But if you make uſe of our new Invention mentioned in the Diſtilling of Corn, you ſave all this trouble: The manner of bringing theſe into *Low Wines*, *Proof Goods*, and *Rectified Spirits*, will be deſcribed in its proper Place.

Now as to Foreign Wines and their Lees, 'tis by us obſervable, that the former being well Fermented and become fine and generous, will give ſo noble a Spirit in Diſtillation, that we highly doubt whether a Pint thereof may be got amongſt all the *Brandy Merchants* in *England*; and becauſe their *Baſis* may be ſold in Foreign parts at a greater price, than when Diſtilled; their uſual way therefore is to Diſtil ſuch Wines, as will not keep the Year about without roping or turning ſowre, or ſuch as are ſmall and defective, in in compariſon to what they are at other Vintages, wherefore we conceive that moſt Brandies are made ſuch Years, as are wet and cold, ſo that the Fruit of the Vine, or Grapes are not for want of the bounteous or friendly Raies of the Sun brought to their true Maturity; from whence only proceed the richneſs and fragrancy to the Wine; for thereby only is the Specificated Sulphur brought forth apparently in its Genuine Nature: Now what Nature doth not perform, they endeavour to ſupply by Art, *ſc.* by ſtumming of them, bringing them by an Artificial heat into a ſtrong Fermentation; and to give Savours, they often uſe the Tincture or Eſſence of appropriated Herbs; and being fine or fined by Glaſs, they rack them off for Sale; concerning which Brewing of Wines, there is no Nation that uſeth it more than the *Dutch*; for altho' in *France* they generally buy the ſmalleſt priſed Wines, new and rough, yet by their ſweets, and perfumes, do they bring and advance them to a conſiderable Price: And theſe alſo thus managed give a very good and pleaſant Spirit or Brandy; being at all times fit for Diſtillation; but that Spirit drawn from the Lees will not by far be ſo pleaſant, as this from the Wines, altho' both out of one and the ſame Cask, as will be ſhown hereafter; therefore paſſing this by here, we ſhall come to ſhow the way of ordering *Low Wines* and *Lees*, which is thus:

You must add to your *Lees* as much warm Liquor as will dissolve them, and then with *Stum* and warmth, or the common Ferment, bring them into Fermentation, and if thick, you may press out the Moisture, and Distil it: But in the Viniferious Countries they mix small, new, and other decayed Wines there-with, and so bring them into Fermentation with some other small addition of Liquor, and then Distil them. So that it is from these mixtures that the Violet, Rasberry, and other pleasant tastes proceed: For as the Ingenious *Glauber* saith, the *Juice of Grapes is nothing else but a sweet Salt, which by Fermentation becomes more Tart; nay, indeed more sowre as its Invisible, Vital and Internal Spirituality hath its more volatile particles exhausted*; but seeing we have more largely treated of Savours in the *Chapter of Rectification*, we shall omit it here, and proceed to the last Head.

The Fermentation of Herbs is to be considered in a twofold respect, *sc.* either as they are worked *per se* by a common Ferment; or by Sugar and Honey; *per se* is when the Herb, Flower or Berry, is bruised in a large Wooden, or Alablaster Mortar, with a Wooden Pestle, and then warm Liquor, or Water poured thereon, and the Ferment or Yeast added sufficient to stir it up or quicken it so, as to bring it into a true and perfect Fermentation; *By Sugar or Honey is*, as you Distil from the Herb its Juice in a cold Still to which, being put in a convenient Vessel, you add Herbs, Fruits or Flowers, well bruised, and

and to every Gallon of Liquor a Pound, two, three, or four of Sugar or Honey, as you will have it in strength; then being stirred well together, let them be covered close and warm; and let them stand till they Ferment, work, froth and flower, and smell very fragrant, and become fit to Distil; and if occasion requires this Fermentation may be promoted by some of the precited Fermentatives. Observe that if you work roots either of these ways you must slice them thin before you put them in.

Thus have we run through these six Heads, in which is comprehended all that is needful to be treated of concerning Fermentation, only we think it requisite to add these following Rules, **First**, *That in all things, that are to be wrought by Fermentation, the whole mixture must be well united*; **Secondly**, *That the Back must be temperately set*; **Thirdly**, *That you must add a convenient quantity of Yeast or Ferment, and keep them warm*: All these must be diligently weighed, and accurately observed, if ever you intend to exalt your materials to the desired end; concerning which you shall hear what the famous *Radolphus Glauber* saith, Where he speaks of the defects in Fermentation; *the which he says sometimes proceeds from too much cold, or hot Water put in, or the Vessels not being well covered, by which means the cold Air is let in, whence the Fermentation is hindred, and consequently the Distillation of the Spirit; for by the help of Fermentation the burning Spirit of the Vegetables is set at liberty, without which it can-*

not be done: Also the Distillation is hindred by too much haste, as well as by too much delay; for if you begin to Distil before the time, viz. *Fermentation not being yet perfected, you shall have but few Spirits; wherefore also the better part is, by many that are unskilful, cast to the Swine, but without any great loss, if the matter were Malt; because that Swine are fed therewith: but not so if other Vegetables were the matter of the Distillation: Also too much slowness where the Matter begins to be sowre before it be Distilled, yields very few Spirits, that which often happens whilest Herbs and Flowers,* &c *are out of Ignorance left in Fermentation three, four, five, or more Weeks, before they be Distilled; for the greatest part of the Spirit is then turned to Vinegar, which would not be so very ill done, if so be these Men knew how to Clarifie the Remainders, and turn it into Vinegar, that nothing thereof might be lost; for the Vinegars of Herbs, Flowers, Seeds and Roots are not to be contemned. And so oftentimes (a thing to be lamented) the better parts, if they be Spices and Precious things, is lost.*

The Matter of the Distillation, and other choice things, as Seeds and Herbs are cast away with loss; wherefore for Admonition sake, I was willing to add such things, that the Operators may have an opportunity to consider the Matter a little more profoundly with themselves, or at least of learning the Art of Distilling from Country Men, who do not suffer their Malt to Putrefie, grow Sowre or Mouldy, before they fall upon their Distillations; but presently Fermentation being made (the third or fourth day) begin their Distillation.

ſtillation. Which we ſhall now come to treat of, and firſt of bringing them into *Low Wines.*

For the making of which you muſt obſerve two things; the firſt is, that in all things, which are Liquid, as Beer, Cyder, *&c.* you muſt put your before deſcribed Pump into the Back in which it is, directing your Spout to that Still which you deſign to charge; and let one Hand Pump, and another pair of Hands Row up, that ſo the Bottom may come into the Still, and when filled ſo high as the upper Nails, let down your Head on the Still; but put not the Beck or Noſe as yet into the Worm; for Reaſons hereafter expreſſed; then, the Still being charg'd, proceed to the making of your Fire, which is beſt of Coals or dry Cleft-Wood, and very ſtrong, until it begins to boyl, as a Pot going over; then muſt you ſet the Pipe of the Head into the Worm, and as it begins to drop and run a ſmall ſtream into the Can, then immediately muſt you throw damping under the Still, which is, the Aſhes that fall under your Grate and kept wet for that end, for if you ſhould not do ſo, it would boyl over into the Worm, and ſo ſtop and foul the ſame; and having proceeded thus far, your Still being in a good Temper, you muſt begin to lute all faſt with a Paſte made of Whiting and Rie-flower: you muſt exactly lute round the Neck of your Still, and by ſo doing you will keep in that Breath, in which is the Spirit; and as you have paſted the Neck, ſo muſt you alſo paſte the Pipe and Worm, wherein it goes; that is to ſay, ex-

actly

actly to close the Joint: You must also observe so to govern your Fire, that you bring your Still to work so, as that the Stream may run the bigness of a large Goose or Turkey Quill; and being thus brought to work, it must be continued till all the strength is off, and what runs is a stinking Flegm; thus are you to proceed in your first Extraction, the second shall be shown hereafter.

As to the other thing, which is to be observed, it is in the Distilling of those things, which are not pressed forth from their Corporiety; but thick and thin must all go into the Still together; and this generally will Cake, although you take all the care you can to stir it before it works; by which means we have known the Bottom of a New Still burnt out; which to prevent, as we have done in our tryals, you must observe, that in making your Still two Inches above the turning, and just even with the closure of the Brick-work, you must have your Still turned with a very large Verge, and exactly hammer'd for the upper part to shut in, which must be proportioned round up, as in other Stills, with a Neck exactly fit for the Head, on which you must place two Rings, just opposite one to another, that so at any time upon occasion it may be easily lifted off, to which Verge you must fit a very strong Iron Hoop, the upper part of which must have three strong Rings in it, that so upon occasion a Rope may be fastned to it; to the under part you must lace or brace on your container, which must come

within

within two or three Inches of the Bottom, as alſo within two Inches of every ſide; then place your Hoop on the Verge, and charge your Still, the Corporiety will be therein received, and the Liquor will paſs to fill up the Vacancy; then ſhut down the Shoulders of your Still, and lute faſt with a Paſte made of *Calx Vive* and Whites of Eggs, or fine Flower and Sand, or thick well boiled Starch and Sand: Let down your Head, but you muſt not yet put the Noſe into the Worm, but make a good Fire, as you were before directed, and ſo cauſe your Liquor to boyl, and before it works great part of the *Wild Gaſs* or unruly Spirit will go off inviſibly, as much indeed as can be expected, except your Liquor had been decocted and cooled in: Now as the Beck, Noſe, or end of the Pipe begins to drop, you muſt put it into the Worm and Lute faſt, as before directed, as alſo the Neck of the Stills, and your Still being brought to work, you muſt in all things proceed in the Extracting your *Low Wines*, as before laid down in the firſt Obſervation: And this alſo is to be Noted, that ſome Malt, Grain, and Fruits will in the beginning run off a Can, two, or three of Proof Spirit, and then it generally runs long: Others ſometimes runs not at the beginning ſo fully Proof, and yet will yield indifferently well. Thus your *Low Wines* being Diſtilled, you let them lye ten or fourteen Days, to enrich themſelves; for in that time they get by lying, and ſome think that if they lie longer they loſe, as alſo *Proof*

Spirits,

Spirits, except they lie very warm: But however they may, as we have found by experience, be so order'd, as that they may be the more mellowed, and better themselves thereby. These Rules being sufficient for the Extracting all kind of *Low Wines*, and the more especially, if you make use of our curious Invention, before described, for that by it these benefits will accrew; First, you are not troubled with the moving, stirring or rowing your matter in the Still; Secondly, you need not fear you Still's being burnt, or your Wines getting any adustion or evil Tang, for they will come over sweet, pleasant and fragrant; Thirdly and Lastly, you have this advantage, that you may remove the Shoulders of your Still, and fasten a Rope in the Iron Hoop, and by means of a Pully lift your matter at once out, which may be received into a Cowel and born away; and the Wash let out the common way; and if your matter be either Wheat or Barley, the Grains, though they have been in the Still, will be very good Food for Cattle or Swine. Note, that after this method, only using a Tin-pan made fit for the Verge, and an Inch or two of vacancy between, whereby to put in the Water, may you have an Artificial *Balneum* for rectifying your Spirits. We shall now proceed to the second Extraction, which is thus;

Take two or three Cans of Water, put them into your Still, and a small handful of Salt; and charge your Still with *Low Wines* to a convenient height: let down your Head, and

and give Fire; then put your Beck into the Worm, and gradually proceed till all is over; the which you may know by the weakness of that which comes.

Observe. You may also use a small Portion of some Herb, which hath a proper Signature with the Vine: And it is a general Custom among the *Distillers*, in order to make their Spirits hot, strong, and fiery in the Mouth, to use *Spanish* Grains, which are sold by the *Druggists*, which do accomplish their end; but with little other advantage to the Spirit: Therefore do we reject it, tho' a thing so much practised, seeing more agreeable and pleasant ways are easily to be found. Now we shall reveal one thing more, which will be helpful to the *Distiller*, which is, in taking away part of the gross Sulphur, from whence much of the Evil Tang proceedeth; and 'tis thus: Take a pound of Wool, wash it exceeding clean, and dry it, and with a Loop hang it in the Head of the Still, in which the Oleous parts ascending, will be insorbed; and when the Operation is over, wash clean, dry, and keep it for the like service: Having thus finished the second Extraction, we think it not amiss to show what quantity of *Low Wines*, *Proof Goods* and *Fine Spirits* may be Extracted from a Quarter of Malt.

You must know, that in the first place, 'twill make about fifty Gallons, or something more than three Barrels of Wash, which in the first Extraction will make thirty two, thirty four, or thirty six Gallons of *Low Wines*; and

and these, if you let them lie, will in the second Extraction yield eleven or twelve Gallons of *Proof Spirit*; nay sometimes (thro' the goodness and richness of the Malt) thirteen; especially if in the second Extraction you add some Water into the Still; which in the third Extraction we count, if truly Proof, lose not many Gallons in a Tun.

Note also, the *English* receive their *Low Wines*, *Proof* and *Fine Goods* in Cans; but the *Dutch* object against this way, saying that it is disadvantageous; because the Spirit is exhausted through the Magnetick or Attractive Property of the Air; therefore they place large receiving Vessels, their full height or more in the Ground, so as to place thick Boards over them, in which they have two Holes; the one for a Funnel to receive the *Low Wines* or *Proof Goods*; the other to put in an Hand-Pump, to Pump them out when they please; which indeed is very commodious, not only for the Reasons mentioned, but also because the Still may be set lower (a Funnel requiring not so large a space or height as a Can) whereby it may be the better and easier commanded.

Thus having run through what was promised in this Chapter, we shall here conclude the same, and pass on to Rectification.

CHAP. II.

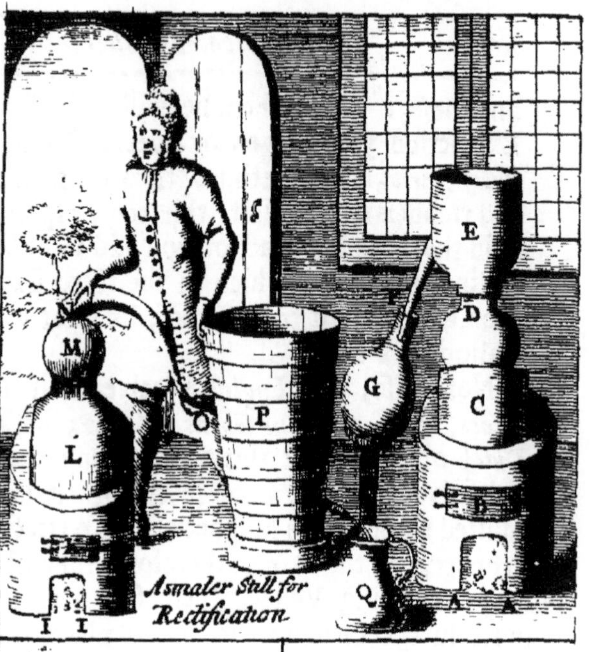

I I the Ash hole
K the Fire place
L the body of the Still
M the Head
N the entering of the Crane nose
O the joyning of the nose therof to the Worme
P the Worme Tubb
Q the Can

The Common Alimbeck wherein small quantityes of Waters are drawn

AA the Ash hole
B the Fire place
C the body of the Still
D the joynt whereat the Head shuts into the Body
E the Cooler containing water to refrigerate the Spirits
F the joyning of the Receiver to the beck of the Alimbeck
G the Receiver

Place this Figure before chap II in page XXX.

CHAP. II.

Wherein we shall Treat of Rectification in General, and also of those **Mediums** *by which 'tis best performed, so as to make Excellent Stuff and Artificial Brandies.*

IN the former Chapter we have Treated of all things necessary, as an Introduction to the Art; so in this we shall now come to speak concerning the Perfection, Corallary and Top-Stone of the same, to wit, that of *Rectification* and making of *Good Stuff* and *Artificial Brandies*, concerning which there is so great a noise about Town, and yet we are all too deficient in this point, altho' in our former Impression, I gave some general Rules for the advancing of this Doctrine, and I hope it had its good Effect among the Industrious, in that we see *Artificial Brandies* brought to a far greater Perfection within these ten Years than in Ages before, yet we are still wanting in the Exaltation of Malt Spirits to that degree, which is desired, *viz.* to give it the true Flavour of Natural Brandy.

'Tis true, *RadolphusGlauber* testifies in *Part.* 1. *pag.* 57. that it is to be perform'd, where he says, " The difference of Malt, by reason " whereof it yields better or worse beer and " Spirit, consists for the most part in the

" Pre-

" Preparation thereof: For being made after
" the Vulgar way it retains its Taste, where-
" fore it can't yield good Stuff nor good Beer,
" which is observed by very few; wherefore
" they could not draw good Spirit out of
" Corn, but such as Savours of the Taste and
" Smell of the Malt, which is not the fault of
" the Corn, but of the Artificer, not opera-
" ting aright in the Preparation of his Malt in
" Distillation and Rectification; for if it
" were prepared aright in all things, Corn
" yields a very good Spirit, not unlike to
" that, which is made out of the Lees of
" Wine, in Taste, Odour and other Vertues;
" which Art, although it be not known to
" all, yet it does not follow that it is im-
" possible.

Now seeing we have so clear a Testimony from so good an Author, concerning the Verity of this, we ought not in honour to question its Authority, but rather impute our deficiency in this Point to the want of that Knowledge enjoyed by him, and therefore let us seriously inquire wherein our defect lies: For certain, it must chiefly consist, either in the manner of ordering the Grain, whether it is to be brewed into Wash or Mash, or to be distilled from protuberated Corn, as the *Dutch* and *Glauberian* way is, or else in some defect in Fermentation, by which the sweet Balsamick part of the Corn is not broken, so as to send forth its Spirits, which is very difficult, seeing that consists in a Gummosity; or otherwise in the want of a due

Medium

Medium to Rectifie from; for that we ſee whatſoever Art we uſe, Malt Spirits are very defective of the true Flavour and Tangue of Brandy, and if theſe are by an Art given it in the Rectification, yet lying a while by, they are loſt again, and the Spirit returns to its old Hogo; ſo that a compleat and ample Knowledge of this ſecret is much to be deſired; and therefore I ſhall give you ſome Hints from Experience, wherein this defect lies, and in which of the three Heads it chiefly depends, as a Particular, or as a General, in the whole.

I ſay it is a Defect in the Whole, for in the firſt Place, if the Grain is not ſo wetted, as to give forth the greateſt part of its Tincture, you cannot expect a pleaſant Spirit; neither if that Tincture be not well fermented and broken, ſo as to imbody the Spirit with its richeſt Sulphur, it will not hold; nor indeed can it obtain a Vinous Flavour, but from Vinous Roots.

As to the Firſt. I do, above all others recommend the Diſtilling of Spirits from protuberated Corn, if the *Engliſh* would but be perſwaded to follow the *Dutch* Example in this Caſe: The Fermentation is a principal Defect, for that we ſee the Waſh left after Diſtillation will, being evaporated and brought to a Slimy Conſiſtence, and then precipitated with the *Alcaly of Tartar*, give a Gummy Rob ſweet and pleaſant, like the ſtrong Elixeration of Malt in Worts, ſo that 'tis plain, that the ſweet *Sulphur* of the Malt is not brought up, and therefore as *Glauber* ſays, *The beſt part of it is given to the Swine*

D It

In Rectification also it is impossible to give it a Vinous Flavour, but by that which has the Nature of a Vinous Sulphur in it; and I make no doubt, but that *Glauber* living in a Viniferous Country, had a *Medium* proper and agreeable at a reasonable Rate to Rectifie from, which we cannot so readily come by here· But we to supply this Defect, use a Rectifying Bag, and some are so abusive to the Health of Mankind as to use *Copperas* therein; others the *Colcothar* of *Aqua Fort* and *Vitriol*; others more wary, use *Nitre*, *Common Salt* and *Chrystals* of *Tartar*, to imbibe the Evil Sulphurs; then to give it a Vinous Taste, they use Herbs and Roots, as *Bay-leaves*, *Mugwort*, *Clary*, *Orrice*, *Pellitory* of *Spain*, *Tamarinds*, *Nettle* and *Thistle Roots*, and many others: But not to the desired Effect; for either they are defective in the right *Pondus*, in that they may be readily over dosed, or else in the due Composition; so that 'tis no difficult matter to know a Pipe or Hogshead of Malt Spirits by its own Name, wherever it lies, altho' there be added in a quantity of *Spiritus Nitri Dulcis*, to give it a Flavour: 'Tis true, the Product of the Goosberry and Syder, and Molasses Goods are brought to an excellent degree of Perfection by mean Artificers or ordinary Operators, so is the Product of Wheat Grain; therefore the whole business of Art is to better the Product of Barley, Buck Wheat, and to mend some defects in the Products of *Rice*, which is called *Rack*, and those of the common *West-India Rum*; and in this I shall contribute what

in

in me lies, for the Benefit of the Industrious, and peradventure may give them some hints, which may yield a Glimmering to the very Truth it self.

I must confess I have sometime doted on the Herb *Scarlea* and *Clary*, but I have not now so great a dependence on Herbs, as on the Product of the Vine; for *Glauber* has at once given a Hint to the Mystery in *Part.* 1. *pag.* 159. where he says, "If any Man will give this "Brandy a Rellish, like that made of the "Lees of Wine, then he must rectifie it upon "the Lees of Wine: For this way by the Oil "of Wine, which is plentiful among the "Lees, he acquires his Ends, and in all things "he may use this instead of that.

But some may make two Objections against this. The first is, "That we have not "Wine Lees enough in this Land, to supply "our want, such great draughts of Malt Spi-"rits being vended. The Second is, That "those rectified from the Lees cannot possibly "be so sweet, as those which are drawn "from pure Wines, because those Lees are "cloathed with Adustion, and so will readi-"ly burn in the Still, or at least give a "stronger Smack, than what is simply drawn "from pure Wines: In answer to these, I say, That they are not comparable to those drawn from rich and generous Wines; but may have some resemblance to those drawn from Vinous Roots of a more inferiour Nature, and especially from the Lees, although Fermented with Molasses, for these being expoſed to the Fire, more than clear Liquors are, will for certain carry ſome Tangue of their Aduſtion with them; whereas on the other hand, Malt Spirits being already brought to ſome Maturity, and then rectified from Lees, theſe Lees may be ſo order'd by the Artiſt, as that they may give the Spirit no ill Tangue; for 'tis obſervable, in the Rectification, the Spirit will only ſuck out the Volatile, Sulphureous and Pleaſant Parts, as is evident in this: If thoſe Lees, from whence you have drawn your Spirits, be afterward Fermented, and then again Diſtill'd, they will yield but little quantity of Spirit, and that deficient in its Flavour, ſo that 'tis evident, there is a difference between Magnetical Attraction and violent Diſtillation, the one bringing up only the Homogenous Parts, and the other ſending off the more Groſs with the Volatile ones; and yet more, if the Spirits you uſe are ſweet and pleaſant, and the *Angel* by Art ſeperated from its Impurities and Terrene *Faces*: Therefore to ſupply both defects, I ſhall lay before you the *Percipiolum* of *Tartar*, publiſhed by *Glauber*, *Part.* 2. *pag.* 139. by which you may make excellent Wines and artificial Brandies. The Receipt is as follows:

" ℞, White or red Tartar (for both " of them being well mundified, are as good " one as the other) diſſolve it in Water, and " ſeparate all its groſs Sulphur, by a certain " precipitating Matter: This impurity abid- " ing in the Water is to be ſeparated from " the precipitated Tartar, by pouring out the

" the Water, the which (Tartar) remains in
" the Bottom like a Snowy Sand, and is to be
" well purged by reiterated Washings with
" Water, so long until (all the Impurities
" being well separated) the Powder it self be-
" comes like to the white Snow. He further
" adds, that this may be so highly exalted, as
" to be associable to Gold: But the Knowlege
" of a Matter precipitating Tartar is not easie
" to be attained to, without which it will ne-
" ver suffer it self to be precipitated and
" Purged: 'tis an hard thing to find, but
" he that knows it, it renders him all his La-
" bour facile and easie: Any impure Tartar,
" whether it be white or red, may be so wash-
" ed in one or two Hours space, and so purg-
" ed, that (losing nothing save its *Faces*) it
" will become most white, and much more
" apt for many Operations. These make
" such fine Spirits of Wine, without any vio-
" lent Distillation, that those Spirits, added
" to Water, will make good Wines, if you
" again add in the depurated Tartar: You
" may also see what he further says in *Part.* 2.
pag. 59. *and Part.* 1. *pag.*292.

Now if you cannot obtain this *Tartar*, then learn the right Use of the *Salt* of *Tartar*, and its *Crystals* in a right *Pondus*, and be sure you do not over-dose it: This is a most excellent *Medium*, which does not only make Spirits sweet and pleasant, but also gives them a Vinous Flavour, and is a Great Secret; for if you know rightly how to work, you may thereof (with the Addition of a small quantity of the

Chrystals) make a perpetual *Mineral:* It's no wonder that Taste and Flavour should proceed from Salts, seeing they have a Sympathy with the Signature of every specificated Sulphur, from whence the Spirits are prepared, which generous Nature will preserve what in her lies, to the utmost Iliad in its fragrancy; but strong Savours either come from the Violence of the Fire or Adustion, so that the Fault is not to be ascribed to Nature, but to the Ignorance of the Operator, seeing the same thing may happen to such, even on the choicest Products of the Vine; as we see *Rum* gets its strong Tangue by the fluffenliness of the Operators, often using the Remains of their Distillations or Wash on the Relicks of New Cane and Sugar for new beginnings instead of Liquor, with the Addition of crude wood-ashes for Ferments; by which means it is brought to have the strongest Smell and Taste of all Vinous Spirits: Which domineering Qualities come from the grosser Sulphur, united with the grosser Salt, or from Adustion; so that consequently a sweet Spirit will proceed from a pure Sulphur, or such as are made so by pure Salts, and united to them in the Act: And so here is no fear of Adustion, for the pure and incombustible part preserves it, therefore it is the great Business of Art, to bereave all sorts of ill savour'd Spirits, of their evil Tangue, and bring them as free from Taste as Water, retaining only their fiery and spiritual Power, and then to introduce what Flavour is most agreeable; and I know none more

more near to that of the Vine, than what may be done by a certain Preparation of Wheat Corn, especially if in the Rectification, a body of pure Salts be put in the Still, with a convenient quantity of Water, that they may have room to cleanse themselves, and to be washed from their foulness, as a Leper from his Leprosie; for those Salts receive and give in the Rectification; they may be said to receive, in that they magnetically attract the Aquosites and Impurities, and also at the same time give forth into the Spirit a pleasant Flavour from the Internal Sulphur.

But by the way you are to observe, there is a great difference in the Use of Salt; for it is twofold; one is rectifying the Spirits through their Bodies in the Still, and the other is their Use in the Cold, by which they perform the same Work, seperating all Impurities without external Fire; which latter, being wrought by a simple Intention, in Nature, excels the former; for all Impurities are gone before they come in the Still, but in this they agree, in both Operations, whereas they rob the Spirits of something, they add something again of their own Nature, by which the Spirits are exalted: I'll give you an Example of this in the following Receipt.

'℞, Pure *Indian Peter* and *White Tartar*, of each a Pound: The best *Yellow Sulphur*, half a Pound, and being finely powder'd and mixed together, you may with a red hot Iron fire them, and when they will burn no more, melt them well in the Fire,

 'and

'and when cold, pour them out into a Mortar,
'and pulverize them very fine immediately,
'or else they will magnetically attract *the*
'*Air, and so not easily admit of being powder'd*:
These forthwith put into a Glass, and pour thereon two quarts of high Proof Spirits, such as you would bereave of their smell, and put them into a cold Place for four or five Days, remembring to shake them twice or thrice a Day, then filter them through a Cap-paper or Filter, and draw off two third parts by Distillation in *Baln. Mariæ*, and so have you your own Spirit again, but of a wonderful pleasant Taste and Smell, far above the former, altho' no Herbs are as yet added; and tho' this at first appearance may not seem to you a thing of Profit; yet it carries with it in its Demonstration such great Truths, as will confirm not only the nature and difference of those, being so wrought, but also the possibility of meliorating or bettering such things as are not drawn from the Products of the Vine, its Profits may also hereafter be considerably discerned, but in all this here is our Mishap, that we are forced to be beholding to foreign Lands for their Product, as Wine, Lees, Tartar, Chrystals, Salt, Nitre, *&c.*

Let us now therefore leave them, and see whether this great business of Art cannot be supplied from the Products of our own Land, I mention this to stir up the Minds of the Ingenious to a diligent search of that, which being obtained will abundantly recompence them

them for their time and labour spent about it; because Nature has blessed this Island with the plentiful Production of one Matter, which is the desire of all true Artists, for a compleat Knowledg of this, supplies all these defects.

The Antient Philosophers testifie, that there is one matter of a Mineral Birth, containing the first *Ens* and Seed of all Metals, which when truly prepared and ripen'd by long Decoction and Conjunction of due Agents and Patients, all Heterogenieties being seperated, and the Homogeneous parts concreted and specificated to a *Metalick Ens*, will then transmute all imperfect Metals into vendible *Sol* and *Lune*: Why then may not the true *Spagyrist* by the help of this Universal Fountain take off the drowsie Nature of *Saturn*, or Spirit of Barley, or the Airy Nature of *Jupiter*, or the Spirit of Fruits, and bring them into that friendly one of *Venus* and the Sun, to which the Vine belongs; seeing the Possibility of Transmutation is by the most pregnant Wits of this Age believed; there is hardly any one, that pretends to any thing in Art, but will argue for the same, and there have been given such undeniable Demonstrations of its Verity, that we think it an impossibility that any reasonable Man should at this time of day doubt thereof, neither indeed have they the least cause to scruple this of Meliorating Spirits.

The easiness of its Performance, I set forth in my former Edition by that Similitude, where I say, 'tis no difficult matter to take the Garments off a poor Man's Back, and to cloath him with richer, as also by the Exam-

ple

ple of casting Elder Flowers into well decocted Mead, whereby it is made like Wine made from the Apian or Muskadine Grape; also how that vulgar *Venus* and *Antimony* will cloath pale Faced *Sol* with a deeper and more beautiful Garment: All which shew, that there is a possibility of bettering Spirits by Rectification; and I know experimentally, that there be some Salts proceeding from the foresaid Universal Matter, which will prepare the *Colcothar* of *Venus* and *Common Sulphur* into a most excellent *Medium* for Rectification; nay, the Matter in it self being exalted and brought into a sweet Salt, will then perform Wonders; for this is that Salt I formerly call'd in my other Edition, the *Chaos* of *Mars* and *Venus*, and in the Preface to *Chymicus Rationalis*, the *Vitriol of Mars and Venus Philosophical*, as being that Chrystalline Lake, a Concentration of all the pure *Effluviums* of the Universal Spirit, brought to a corporal or bodily Form, yet nevertheless acts like a Spirit, and hath power to alter things for the better, which in this Case cannot properly be call'd a Transmutation of Form, for that is a changing of one kind into another: but this is a Melioration or Alteration from an indifferent to a better State; that is, it will seperate Impurities, gross Sulphurs and stinking Flegms, from whence the nauseous Smells and Tastes do proceed, and more especially if they are made Fœtid by being burnt in the Still, and render them fragrant and pleasant; it does not perform these good Offices only on

Spirit

Spirit of Wine, but also on Wines themselves, even in all things the Artist can desire to a superlative Degree; for if Wines are kill'd or dead by their Spirit being separated by Distillation, the said Spirit being return'd to its Salt and Flegm, and brought to a knew Fermentation by the *Medium* of this Salt, they will then assume their own generous Nature and Goodness again; for this Reason I have call'd this Great *Medium* **Sal Panaristos**, of whose Original and Parts I have given some hints in the second Part.

Now for the obtaining of these things, you must search with indefatigable diligence, for as **Solomon** says, *the diligent hand makes rich*, which may be understood of Knowledg as well as Substance; seeing that he himself prefers Wisdom and Understanding, before all the Riches and Glory of this World; saying, *Kings and Princes must come and throw down their Crowns and Scepters before it*; how can any Man be said to excel another, if he have not some Gifts above him, and a Practical Knowledg in that, of which the other understands nothing; but into this Part must every Man enter by his own self labour, and unceessant seeking and knocking until divine Providence, through his Perseverance, shall open it unto him; for we can neither lay, nor yet think of any Limitations in this case, but conclude, that what we have written is sufficient for any rational *Genius* to receive Information, and make Improvement by: therefore I shall pass by the *Theory*, and come to shew the *Practic Part* in Rectification.

Now

Now in Rectification you are to take any Proof Spirits, and charge your Rectifying Still to the Nails or two thirds, let it be greater or lesser, whether Barrel or Hogshead, according as your work is, if you use Herbs or gross things to Rectifie from, then tye them up in a bag, which they call a Rectifying-bag, and hang it in a string about three Inches from the bottom to preserve it from burning, but if you use Salts cast them loose into your Still with a little *Clary* or *Orrice*, or what you think fit, clap on your Head and Lute fast with a Paste made of Whiting and Rie meal, and gently draw off your fine Goods.

You must be very cautious of Fire and Candles, especially where there is any breaking out of fume, least it should take fire, and so do much mischief, for this reason is Rectification abundantly more dangerous than drawing *Low Wines*; therefore be not too hasty, but proceed warily and moderately, and govern it so, that the stream may not run above the bigness of a large Crow quill, or at most of a small Goose one; and if your Still be large, so that your Worm Fat heat, then you must be mindful to cool it; and observe that you let it not run too long, for the latter part of your Spirit will be apt to carry some illSavour with it, to the great detriment of the former; therefore let that be saved apart, the first for Brandies, the latter to be again Rectifyed so as to fire Gunpowder, and then it may be used for Varnishes, or else it may serve for some Compound Waters

Now

Now to know when all the Spirituality is over, you may proceed thus: Take a Taster of that which runs in the left hand, and a lighted Candle in the right, throw it upon the Neck or Head of the Still at work, immediately putting the Candle thereunto; and if it takes fire and burns, you may proceed; otherwise your Operation is at an end, this is the common Proof, but I usually judge of it by the Taste, because Experience has shewn me, that when it would not fire, it would nevertheless yield some Gallons better than some *Low Wines*.

If in this Tryal of Rectification, all things do not succeed to your Expectation, proceed to a second, or third; sometimes with one sort, sometimes another sort of Herbs and Salts, until you obtain the Vinous Taste, and have a clean Spirit and then be content; for that there is a diversity in Brandies made from different sorts of Wine, as that of *Spanish* and *French*, for the first proceeds from a Wine, wherein there is all the Sweetness imaginable, being endued with many pleasant and grateful *Effluviums*, yet it makes not so good Brandies, as the *Rhenish* and *German* Wines do, neither do either of these make so good as those of *France*; tho these are not endued with that Natural Sweetness, as those are, but are more tart, and yet give the most flavorous and pallatable Brandies, for tho all sweet Wines naturally give a sweet Spirit, yet it follows not, that they are as grateful, as those which are more sharp, so that you are to consider the difference

ference between tart and ſweet, together with the predominancy of the ſpecificated Sulphurs; for from hence comes the different Flavours in Vinous Spirits; for if the ſweet has Predominance with the Flavours of the *Rhinal* ſoyl, then the Violet Taſte is evidently diſcernable; but from the red Mold of *France*, the tart gives the Rasberry Taſte; and theſe again being mixed give neutral and pleaſant Flavours, whoſe difference is eaſily diſcernable by curious Pallats, altho it cannot be ſo exactly compared to what it is moſt like in flavour, ſo many curious ones being intermixed.

You are alſo to obſerve, that clear Wines yield much more grateful Spirits than the Lees, as being freed from *fæces* or Sediments and groſs, fæculent Sulphurs, which corrupt their Sweetneſs; ſo there is a difference between thoſe made from ripe and generous Wines, and ſuch as are from ſowre and unripe ones: Alſo thoſe that are made *per ſe*, do much vary from thoſe made from ſeveral ſorts of Wines thrown in together, the like may be underſtood of their Lees: Many things of this nature might be ſaid, ſeing Nature, the Miſtreſs of things, is ſo bounteous and large in her gifts: but we muſt be forced to omit many things, leaſt this Treatiſe ſhould ſwell too big, wherein we deſign to be as conciſe and compact as may be, and ſo we ſhall now deſiſt from Rectification, and come to give you the way of allaying and colouring.

The

The common allay is by adding Water till you bring it down to *Proof*; but ſome make a ſtrong *Lixivium* of *Calx vive*, and then diſtil the clear Water with an Addition of a few *Chryſtals* of *Tartar*; this they ſay mixes without the leaſt Bubble or white Speck, or ſeeming Precipitation.

To colour it, they generally take a Tincture of *Logwood* and yellow *Saunders*, with ſome of the Spirit, and then add in, what is ſufficient to colour the whole; ſome add broad *Mace*, *Nutmeg* and *Cinnamon*, more or leſs, according to the quantity; others a few drops of *Oyl* of *Cinnamon*, *Cloves* and *Mace*, drop'd into fine Sugar, and then put in with half their quantity of *Ambergreaſe*; but obſerve that all theſe are to be added in ſo ſmall a quantity as not to be diſcern'd, and then let your Brandies lye by to mellow. Let this ſuffice concerning Brandies: We ſhall now come to what remains, as pertinent to be treated of in this Chapter, *viz.* the true way of preparing ſimple Waters and Spirits; ſuch I mean as have no more than the Spirit and one ſingle Herb or *Species*; becauſe in many Caſes, 'tis convenient to have their Vertues *per ſe*.

Of

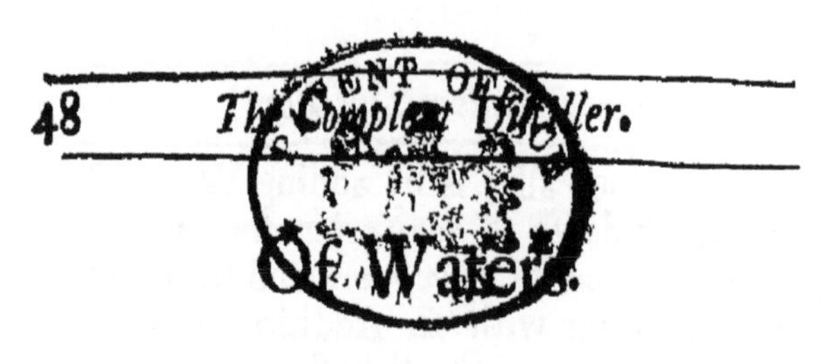

Of Waters.

Aqua Anisi Simplex, *or, Simple Aniseed Water.*

Composition the least.

TAKE of Artificial Brandy, one Gallon, Aniseeds bruised twelve Ounces, put them into the like Alimbeck described in Fig. 3. and in *Balneo* Distil off the fine Spirit, *S. A.* then take two quarts of the Water cleansed by *Calx vive*, Aniseeds bruised four Ounces, and in a cold Still, Distill off something more than a Quart, in which Water gently dissolve on the Embers, twelve Ounces of fine white Sugar, and when cold, therewith allay and dulcifie the Spirits already refined, and so is the Water prepared.

'This Water is an excellent Carminative, 'expelling Wind in the Bowels, and all parts 'of the Body; in brief, it Answers all that 'can be attributed to the Spirit, Tincture, 'Infusion or Decoction of the Seeds. The 'Dose from one Spoonful to three.

Aqua

Aqua Cardamomi Simplex, *or, Simple Cardamom Water.*

Composition the least.

Take of Brandified Spirits one Gallon, Cardamom Seeds one Pound, Operate in all things as in the former; likewise prepare a Syrup, as there directed, with which dulcifie and allay.

'This Water is very prevalent in warming 'and strengthning the Stomack, comforting 'the Vital Spirits, and expelling Wind, car- 'rying with it all the Virtues, that may be at- 'tributed to any other preparation of the Seed. 'The Dose is the same as the former.

After this way may be prepared the Water from most Seeds, as Caraways, Daucus, sweet Fœnil Seeds, *&c.* the which we shall not repeat, seeing their preparation is one with this, and their Virtues to be understood after the same manner: Therefore I shall proceed no further therein, but come to Herbs.

Aqua Cardami simplex, *or, simple Garden Cress-water.*

Composition the least.

Take of Brandified Spirit one Gallon, Garden-Cresses fresh gathered, half a Peck, macerate them in your Alimbeck three days, and then Distill into fine Goods, *S. A.* Also from the Herb *per se* in the cold Still Distill the cold Water, to every three Pound of which, you must add one Pound of fine Sugar, the which dissolve therein, and then therewith allay and dulcifie the Spirit; let it refine, and so is it prepared.

'This Water helps to expectorate and 'raise tough Flegm, destroys Worms, and 'is good against the Yellow Jaundice, and any 'Poison whatsoever, but it is more appropri- 'ated to Men than Women, because 'tis hurt- 'ful to the *Fœtus.* Now *Nasturtium,* or the Herb Cresse common may be worked in all things like this, whose Virtues, as 'tis said, were among the *Persians* esteemed so great, that when from home they eat no other meat, to revive their Spirits.

Aqua Menthæ simplex, *or, simple Mint-Water.*

Composition the lesser.

Take of Brandified Spirit, three Gallons, Mints gathered in their right signature, and gently dried, eight handful, macerate them three days, and then Distill in *Balneo, S. A.* and with the Distilled Water of the Green Herb made in a cold Still, with the same prepara-tion, as before directed, dulcifie and allay.

This

This Water heats the Stomach, and prevents Vomiting, two or three ſpoonfuls being taken as occaſion requires. Obſerve, that by this Rule you may make many other Waters; as Bawm, Angelica, Wormwood, *&c.* being gathered in their prime, and gently dried; and you may proportion them to your Brandified Spirit, more or leſs in quantity, according as you will have your Waters weaker or ſtronger of the Herb: And you muſt alſo obſerve the Nature of the Herbs, for one is abundantly ſtronger than the other, for an handful of Wormwood will go farther than two or three of ſome other Herbs: Now in making your Wormwood-water, we adviſe you not to take the Water made from a cold Still, but that which comes from the Diſtillation of the Oyl, and to every quart thereof add two ounces of Ginger and one of Orrice, and Diſtill again in a cold Still, and then with what quantity of fine Sugar you pleaſe, gently diſſolved upon the Embers, you may allay and dulcifie. As to their Virtues, they ſhall be here omitted, ſeeing 'tis plainly to be conceived, that they contain the Virtues of the ſimple Herb, and all other that can be attributed to any other preparation of this kind: And as to their more exalted Preparations and Virtues, they are treated of more at large in the Chapter of *Powers.*

Aqua Violæ Tricoloris Simplex, *or, simple Hearts-Ease Water.*

Composition the least.

Take of Artificial Brandy one Gallon, Hearts-Ease, in the prime, *&c.* when seeded being gently dried, one pound and a half, put them into your Still, and let them macerate three days, then Distill in *Baln.* into fine Goods, *S. A.* You may allay and dulcifie as before directed, either with their own Syrup, or Syrup of Violets.

Its Virtues. ' 'Tis an excellent Cordial, far ' above any other, for such as are faint and ' weak in the *French*-Pox, also for Fevers, ' Measles, or Small-Pox; and for Agues, ' Convulsions and Falling-sickness; the ' *Ægyptians* highly esteemed of this for Epi- ' lepsies; but we know that this Water is ' good for those that have weak and inflamed ' Lungs, Consumptions, *&c.*

Aqua Raphani Simplex, or, Radish Water Simple.

Composition the lesser.

Take of Brandified Spirits, three Gallons, of Garden Radish fresh gathered, clean washed and sliced, six pound, macerate three days with Mustard and an Onion, and then Distill in in *Balneo. S. A.* You may allay with the cold Distill'd water of Arsmart, and dulcifie with Syrup of Marsh-Mallows, and then let it become fine, and so is it prepared.

Its Vertues. ' 'Tis an excellent Lithontrip-
' tick bringing off Gravel, and provoking
' Urine, it dissolves Clotted Blood and ex-
' pels it; 'tis good in old Coughs, attenua-
' ting gross humours in the Chest; it kills
' Worms, and expels them, it provokes the
' Terms, and gives ease in the Cholick, 'tis
' good for Women after delivery, to help to
' expel the Secundine, and also to prevent
' from Feverish Symptoms; in brief its Vir-
' tue is such, as that it may be safely Admi-
' nistred in Melancholick, Splenetick and
' Scorbutick Diseases: Its Dose is one, two,
' three or four Spoonfuls according to the
' Age and Strength of the Patient.

Aqua Sabinæ Corticis Simplex, *or, Savine Water simple.*

Composition the least.

Take of Brandified Spirit, one Gallon; of the Bark of Savine six ounces, macerate three days and Distill, *S. A.* You need not dulcifie it, nor allay it: ' For 'tis mostly designed for
' washing of Ulcers, either Scrophulous or
' Cancerous, for abating Inflammations and
' dissipating Nodes and Tumours; 'tis seldom
' or never given inwardly, without it be to

'provoke the Menses, or to expel the dead 'Fætus; then the Dose is half a Spoonful, 'or Spoonful in White or Rhenish Wine, 'sweetned with Sugar.

Having laid down these Examples, we shall not insist upon any more of this kind, seeing they are sufficient to show you the Preparation, not only of Seeds, Herbs, Flowers, Roots and Barks; but also of Berries and Spices, and others of the Vegetable Kingdom: We shall in the next Place show you the way of Perfuming them, and then proceed to those of an higher Order, *sc.* Spirits.

The way to Perfume them.

Take of the Sulphurated Spirit of Wine mentioned in the Chapter of Rectification three Pound, Jessamine Flowers half a Pound, Honey Suckle Flowers four ounces, Orange Flowers, or the fresh Pill two ounces, macerate twenty four Hours, and Distill in *Balneo, S. A.* And to the Spirit that comes over add Ambergreese four scruples, Musk two scruples, which being cut small, put them into a Bolthead, Seal them Hermetically, and digest with a very gentle heat till dissolved; the which put in Bottles, with stone stoppers for use.

The manner how, is to add such a quantity to the Waters, as you will have them in strength of the Perfume.

Of

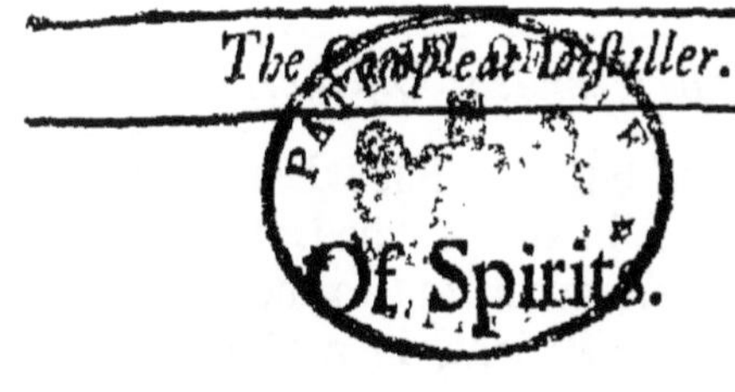

Of Spirits.

Spiritus Salviæ, *or, Spirit of Sage.*

TAKE of Artificial Brandy three Gallons, Sage in its Bloſſom, Prime, and chief Signature, twelve Pound, macerate them for three days, and then Diſtill as long as goodneſs comes; then take ſix or eight pound of freſh Sage, and Diſtill as before: And with freſh Sage ſix pound repeat a third time, carefully preſerving the firſt Gallon that comes, and what comes more you may reſerve for another Operation, to uſe inſtead of Brandy.

Its Virtues. 'Tis one of the greateſt Friends that the Female Sex have, amongſt all the ſingle Concretes in the Vegetable Kingdom, for 'tis prevalent in opening of all Obſtructions, it cleanſes the Blood, provokes the Menſes, cloſes the Matrix, and makes them Fruitful, and very excellent, when with Child, to keep them from miſcarriage: Its general Virtues are for quickning the Senſes and Memory, ſtrengthening the Sinews and Nerves: And therefore good in Apoplexies, Palſies, and Convulſions; nay, ſhould we be particular in every point of its Virtues, we might fill a whole Sheet therewith: This Spirit makes excellent Sage Beer or Wine, an ounce thereof being put

'into a quart of either. But when you take
'the Spirit alone in drops, the Dose is from
'twenty to sixty, according to the Age and
'Strength of the Patient, in a Glass of ei-
'ther.

Spiritus Cochleariæ, *or, the Spirit of Scurvey-Grass.*

Take of Scurvey-Grass, in *June* or *July*, Herbs, Flowers, and all; bruise it well in a large Marble Mortar, and put to every Peck one Pound of Honey, and a little Bay Salt, and let them Ferment two or three days in a cold Cellar; for in a warm place much of their *Crasis* will be lost; which consists in a Volatile Salt, then cram these into your Still as close as ever you can, and pour upon them of the best Æthereal Spirit of Wine, enough only to moisten them, clap on the Head, and Distill all with a very slow fire, it can't be too gentle, therefore in this be very careful; and what comes over first will be the true Spirit of Scurvey-Grass you may proceed by a second Repetition, and then to every Gallon of this spirit add a Pound of its own Seeds or Flowers, and Distill again: And be sure in these Operations you observe to take no more than the high spirit: Now for the remaining spirit in the Still, you must put to it a quantity of decripitated Bay-salt, and Distill as long as it comes Proof; with which you may begin your next Distillation with fresh Scurvey-Grass,

Grass, proceeding as before. This is the true and best way, to prepare the right spirit of Scurvey-Grass. To make it Golden and Purging, we refer you to our *Chymicus Rationalis.*

Its Virtues. ' 'Tis proper in the Scurvey, ' Dropsie or Jaundice, *&c.* which we shall not ' here repeat, seeing we have spoken thereof ' in its proper and genuine Preparation, *sc.* ' that of Powers. The Dose is from thirty ' to fifty Drops according to the Age and ' strength of the Patient.

Spiritus Lavandulæ, *or, Spirit of Lavander.*

Take of Brandified Spirit three Gallons, of Lavander Flowers twelve Pound, Oyl of Salt *per deliquium* two Pound, macerate in a gentle warmth ten or twelve Days, then Distill in *Bal.* as long as goodness comes, in which macerate one Pound of the Oyl of Salt *per se.* and eight Pound of fresh Flowers, and Distill, as before: Lastly, Rectifie from six Pound of Flowers *per se,* and so it is prepared.

Its Virtues. ' 'Tis excellent for all Diseases ' of the Head, as, Megrims, Epilepsies, Con- ' vulsions and Calentures, as also for violent ' and inveterate Head-Achs, here it is a ' Specifick, it is prevalent in fortifying the ' Animal Spirits, and good in the Cholick, ' Strangury and Disentery, the over much ' flowing of Womens Terms, and all other ' Fluxes of Blood. The Dose and manner of ' Administration is as the former. Ob-

Obſerve, after this way is prepared the Spirit of Roſemary, but ſeeing we have at large ſhowed its right and genuine Preparation in Chapter the fourth, together with its Virtues and Uſe, we ſhall omit it here.

Spiritus Angelicæ, *or, Spirit of Angelica.*

Take of Angelica in its right Signature, as much as you pleaſe, pound it in a large Stone Mortar with a Wooden Peſtil, and putting it into your Still, cover it over a Fingers breadth with pure Brandified Spirit, and with a piece of Leaven, let it macerate three or four Days; then Diſtill as long as goodneſs will come; repeat this a ſecond time with freſh Herbs; then to every Gallon of Spirit add of *Spaniſh* Angelica Roots ſliced thin two Pound, and rectifie therefrom; the fine Spirit you muſt reſerve for uſe, and the other may ſerve for a new Beginning.

Its Virtues. '’Tis very prevalent againſt 'all Poiſon, and Infectious corrupted Airs, 'the Peſtilential Fever or Plague, it carries off 'the Venom by Sweat and Urine, and inſen- 'ſible Tranſpiration; it comforts the Heart 'and Vital Spirits, and therefore excellent 'to be uſed by ſuch as are bitten with any 'Venomous or Mad Beaſt whatſoever: ’Tis 'powerful in opening the Obſtructions of the 'Liver or Spleen, bringing down the Terms, 'and expelling the Secundine. The Doſe is 'from one Scruple to three, in a Glaſs of '*Spaniſh* or Rhenish Wine.

Spirit

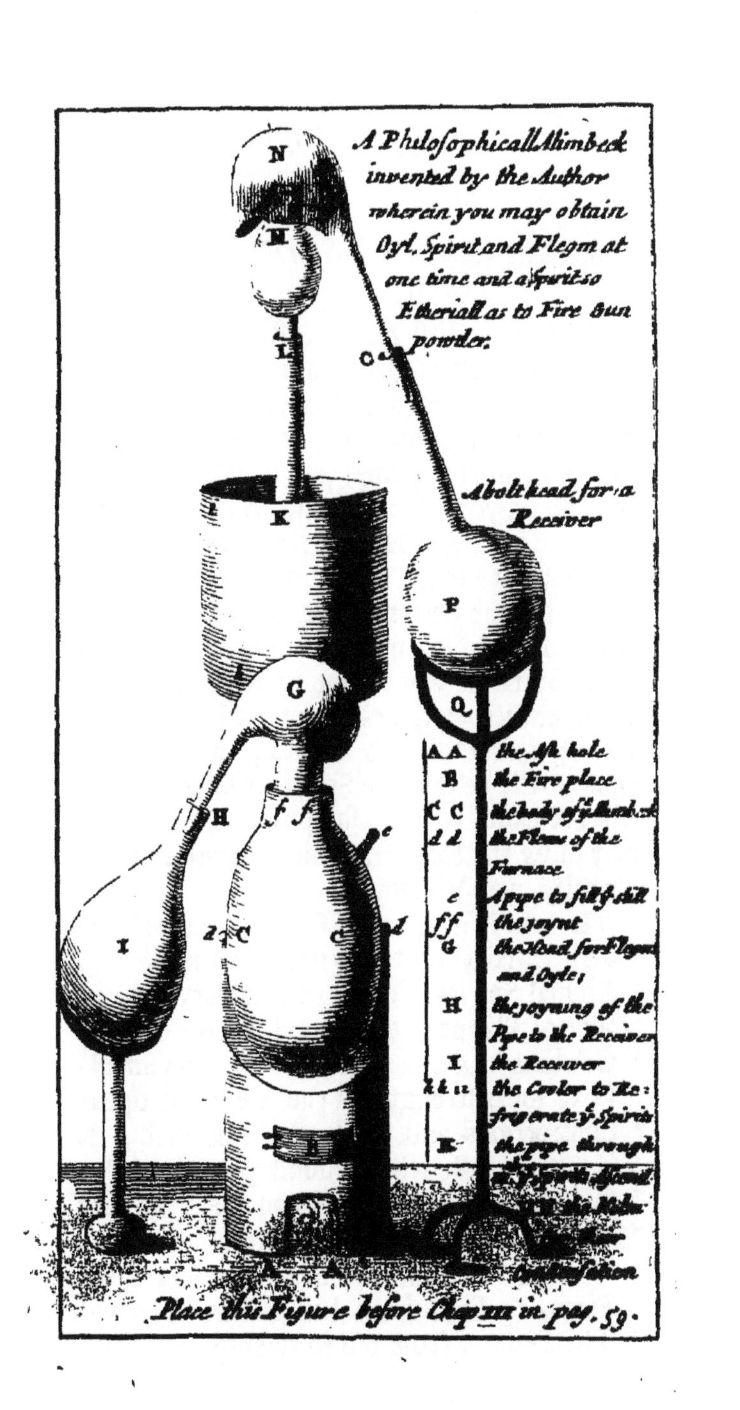
A Philosophicall Alimbeck invented by the Author wherein you may obtain Oyl, Spirit and Flegm at one time and a Spirit so Etheriall as to Fire Gun powder.
N
M
L
O
K
A bolt head for a Receiver
P
G
Q
H
I
C
C
d
e
f f
A A the Ash hole
B the Fire place
C C the body of ye Alimbeck
d d the Flame of the Furnace
e A pype to fill ye still
f f the joynt
G the Head for Flegm and Oyle;
H the joyning of the Pipe to the Receiver
I the Receiver
k k the Cooler to Refrigerate ye Spirits
K the pipe through
Condensation
Place this Figure before Chap XIII in pag. 59.

Spiritus Croci, *or, Spirit of Saffron.*

Take of the best *English* Saffron one Pound, of Malaga Sack a Quart, Honey half a Pound, Chrystals of Tartar four Ounces, let the Chrystals of Tartar be beat very well with the Saffron in a Mortar; then put it into a Glass, and add in your Honey and Wine; lute all fast, and in a gentle heat let them Ferment and macerate ten, twelve, or fourteen days, the longer the better; then take off the blind Head, and add in three Quarts of the Sulphurated Spirit of Wine, put on its Helm, with a proper recipient, being truly adapted, lute all fast, and Distill in *Balneo*; the two first Quarts will be the true Spirit. Observe from what remains with fresh Spirit of Wine, you may draw the Extract, which though small in quantity, yet Virtuous.

The Spirits Virtues. 'Tis an excellent Cordial, fortifying the Vital, Natural, and Animal Spirits; 'tis a great Preservative in time of Plague; 'tis beyond all the cooling Cordials in *England* for Measles and Small-Pox, for it strengthens the Heart, it opens Obstructions and heals the Phthisick, it brings Breath when almost gone, and 'tis said to prolong Life; if you wash the Face with it, mixt with Rose Water, in the time of Small-Pox, and Measles, it preserves the Face and Eyes from being hurt thereby: The Dose is from ten to twenty, and from

'twenty

'twenty to sixty Drops in some Cordial
'Julep, or Wine, as the Patient best
'likes.

Spiritus Dauci, *or, Spirit of Daucus.*

Take of Wild Carrotseed twelve Pound, beat them small, put them into your Still, and add thereunto of the Sulphurated Spirit of Wine three Gallons, of *Mevis* Sugar three Pound, macerate them for ten or twelve days, and then Distill off one half, the which preserve for Spirit; the other half may be run off for fresh Beginnings. You may if you please put it all together on fresh Seeds, and make another Reiteration.

Its Virtues. 'It is a Carminative, breaking and consuming Wind, good in the Gripes and Cholick, Fits of the Mother, provoking the Terms: In fine, 'tis good in the Strangury, Disury, Gravel and Stone, and provokes Urine. The Dose is from thirty to sixty Drops, proper at all times for such as are subject to the forementioned Diseases, but principally when mostly therewith assaulted.

Thus (Reader) have we laid you down examples sufficient for the making of simple Waters and Spirits so that if you have but an ordinary *Genius*, you may arrive to what you desire therein, and if you can't attain to the Art of Distillation by these plain Rules and Precepts contained in this Book, then do we we highly doubt, whether you'll ever be able to attain it, but by Ocular Demonstration; therefore our advice is that you should apply your self to some honest *Distiller*, for you may learn more of him in six Weeks time, than in years by your own Study and chargeable Operations, and therefore count it a considerable Favour, if such an one will be thy Friend; yet have we done here to our utmost to serve you, and according to our twenty Years experience have left nothing deficient, not so much as a Tittle: If you proceed therein *secundum Artem Distillationis*, which is impossible to be delivered in writing, Experience must be the chief Mistriss herein, and as you proceed so, we doubt not of prizing our Labours, which are committed to the World for the Benefit of such as are groaping, as we may say at Noon day for satisfaction therein, but here if you clear your sight, you will discern a small Lamp burning, by the which you may open the Chest to the choicest Mysteries thereof.

I have described all the necessary Stills and Furnaces in their several Figures, so that we shall now proceed to the next Chapter, in which will be laid down all the necessary Waters, that will fully supply the *Distiller* with what may be desired of him for publick Sale.

CHAP. II.

CHAP. III.

In which we shall give you the Composition and way of preparing of **Aqua Vitæ**, *and other rich Cordial Waters, in their greater and lesser* **Pondus**, *stated from the greatest Authority of Art.*

THE Receipts here prescribed derive their Foundation from the best Masters in *Europe*, sc. *German*, *Dutch* and *English*, &c. that have Master-like treated hereof; so that we have been at no small pains, to compare and then compute their differences, thence taking such a *Medium*, as that the subsequent prescriptions may well serve for either; nay, indeed much better than some others extant, for in the first place the exact quantity of the Spirit is mentioned, and in the second the just *Pondus* and quantity of all the Ingredients, even to a Grain: Now as to the first 'tis very convenient and helpful to the young Practitioners in this Art, seeing they may be mistaken in that general term, *Take Proof Spirit what sufficeth*; and so take either too much or too little, and thereby destroy the harmonious flavours of their Waters: so is also the second, for many Grains in a Composition, where various things are named, will amount to Scruples and Drachms, and so make a considerable alteration, especially in such as are prescribed for Physical uses; in in the which we ought to be very cautious, that ſo their virtues may anſwer the Preſcriber's end. Now having given you to underſtand the reaſon, why we have ſtuck ſo cloſe to this Method, *&c.* for it's exactneſs, from whence Superiority proceeds; what remains, as convenient to be treated of in this place, is only to mention the Meaſures, and then go on to the Receipts themſelves: As to the Meaſures, the *Dutch* uſe Cans, Stopes, Small Cans, Pints, Half-pints and Muddikeys: The *Engliſh* Cans, Gallons, Quarts, Pints, Half-pints, and Quarter-pints; the *Dutch* Can is ſix Stopes, and three Stopes are exactly two *Engliſh* Gallons, ſo that their Quarts, Pints, Half-pints, and Quarters are abundantly bigger than the *Engliſh*; but finding the *Engliſh* Can generally to be four Gallons, which exactly make ſix Stopes, which is the ſame with the *Engliſh* Can, we ſhall divide our meaſure thus, into Cans, Half-Cans, and Quarter Cans; which is to be underſtood four Gallons; two Gallons and one Gallon, this the *Engliſh* may compute by their Gallons, and the *Dutch* by their Cans; ſo that neither need to be in any Labyrinth. Now by the way you are to obſerve, that in the following common Waters, a Tun of Proof Spirits will make near a Tun and a half thereof. That is, by help of the ſweets and allays.

Aqua

Aqua Vitæ.

Composition the greater.

Distiller. Take of Strong Proof Spirit four Cans or sixteen Gallons, Anniseeds bruised one pound eight ounces, three drachms, twelve Grains, and adding a Can of Water as advised in Rectification, Distill into fine Goods, or as long as it comes pleasant: If it should be above Proof you may allay it, the way how will be shewn hereafter.

Composition the lesser.

Take of strong Proof Spirit three Gallons, or ¾ of a Can, Anniseeds bruised four ounces, four drachms; and distill into fine goods, as before directed, *S.A.*

Aqua Vitæ.

A second Prescription, and Composition the greater.

Distiller. Take of strong Proof Spirit sixteen Gallons, Anniseeds two pound, Caraway Seeds, Coriander-seeds, *ana.* four ounces; distill into fine goods, *S.A.*

Composition the lesser.

Take of high Proof Spirit three Gallons, Anniseeds nine ounces, six drachms, Caraway Seeds, Coriander Seeds, *ana.* one ounce, one drachm, distill them into fine goods, *S.A.*

P.-worth. 'Tis the manner of the *Dutch* to colour these *Aqua Vitæ's* with Alkanet Root, or Turnsole, which is Linen Rags died Red; their manner is thus: They take a quart of *Aqua Vitæ*, and of either of these four ounces, Musk and Ambergreese, *ana.* grains fourteen or sixteen, or more or less, as they will have it in strength; they stop it close in a Bottle, setting it in a gentle warmth, and then draw off the Tincture, the which, when cold, they add in such quantity to their *Aqua Vitæ's*, as they would have them in height of colour. But the *London Distiller* uses Gilly-Flowers, Roses, Poppy, Sanders, or any of them severally, what sufficeth, and infuses them in *Aqua Vitæ*, or Proof Spirit, till the Tincture be drawn out; then decants the Spirit, and reserve it (close stopt) for use; which is to tinge or colour your *Aqua Vitæ*'s upon occasion, the proportion may be about eight Ounces to one Gallon, or what more or less you think sufficient to answer your expectation: If you add in a little fine Sugar, 'twill not be amiss.

Its Virtues. ' 'Tis an excellent Carmi-
' native, for two or three spoonfuls being
' drank will expel Wind in the Bowels or
' any other parts of the Body; a spoonful

'thereof being taken in any Paroxiſm with 'as much Water, relieves or helps the Pati- 'ent; being alſo very proper for ſuch as are 'weak and faint, through Obſtructions, to be 'taken Mornings.

Aqua Vitæ aurea ſecundum Glauber:

or,

Glauber's *Golden Aqua Vitæ.*

Compoſition the leaſt.

Take of high Proof Spirit, drawn from the aurified Salt, ſpoken of in the Chapter of Rectification, one Gallon, to which add Flowers of the Lilly of the Valley twelve Ounces, red Roſes, Cinnamon, Mace, Cardamums, Burrage, Roſemary, Sage, Lavender, *ana.* half a pound; Ambergreeſe and Musk, *ana.* two, three or four ſcruples, let all theſe Flowers be freſh gathered, and being in the Veſſel with the dried Spices, let them macerate for ten or twelve days, then Diſtill: If you cannot get freſh Flowers, you muſt even content your ſelf with dried ones; but the freſh gather'd would be better, if they can be had.

Virtue. 'This is an incomparable *Aqua 'Vitæ*, and may ſafely be uſed in all ſickneſs 'of the Body whatſoever, and moſt profita- 'ble where the Vital Spirits, Heart and Brain 'want to be ſtrengthen'd. The Doſe is from

'half

'half a ſpoonful or two ſpoonfuls at moſt, as
'occaſion requires. And this being taken in
'caſe of neceſſity, or as ſome illneſs preſents,
'you may eaſily diſcern how far its Virtues
'ſurpaſs other *Aqua Vitæ's.*

Aqua Aniſi, *or, Aniſeed Water.*

Compoſition the greater.

Diſtiller. Take of good Proof Spirit ſixteen Gallons, Aniſeeds bruiſed ſeven pound, eight ounces, ſeven drachms, eight grains. Diſtill into ſtrong Proof Spirit, and then dulcifie with white Sugar ſeven pound, eight ounces, ſeven drachms, eight grains, *S. A.* [**Addition**] of Aniſeeds and white Sugar, *ana.* ſeven pound, eight ounces, ſeven drachms, eight grains, or what is ſufficient to anſwer your end, as you'll have it ſtronger or weaker of the Seeds and Sugar.

Compoſition the leſſer.

Take of ſtrong Proof Spirit three Gallons, Aniſeeds bruiſed one pound, and a half, then diſtill into ſtrong Proof Spirit, and dulcifie it, with white Sugar one pound, and a half [**Addition**] Aniſeeds, white Sugar, *ana.* one pound and a half.

Worth. 'This is an excellent Water
'to ſtrengthen the Stomach, Breaking, Cut-
'ting and Expectorating tough Phlegm, help-
'ing the digeſtive Faculty, giving eaſe and

 'ſtrength-

'ſtrengthning in the Phthiſick or ſhortneſs of
'Breath; it abates wind in the Stomack,
'Bowels and other parts of the Body; and
'therefore proper for ſuch as give ſuck, to be
'taken to the quantity of half an ounce, to
'prevent Wind, which ſucking Children are
'ſo ſubject to.

Aqua Angelicæ, *or, Angelica Water.*

Compoſition the greater.

Diſtiller. Take of high Proof Spirit ſixteen Gallons, Angelica Roots two pound ſix ounces, and a Qr. or Angelica Herb green, eleven pound and a half, Aniſeeds one pound, nine ounces, ſix drachms, ſlice the Roots thin, or bruiſe them and the Seeds; then diſtill into fine Goods, and dulcifie with white Sugar eight pound. [**Addition**] Carraway ſeeds, Coriander ſeeds, *ana.* four ounces, ſix drachms and a half, *Calamus Aromaticus, Zedoary, ana.* ſix ounces and a half, Aniſeeds, Caſſia Lignea, *ana.* half a pound, four ounces and a half, Angelica Root, twelve ounces and a half, or Herb Angelica three pound three ounces, one drachm and a half, white Sugar four pound.

Compoſition the leſſer.

Take of high Proof Spirit three Gallons, Angelica Roots ſix ounces, ſix drachms, or

Ange-

Angelica Herb Green two pound, four ounces, Aniseeds four ounces, seven drachms, slice the Roots thin, or bruise them and the Seeds; then Distill into fine Goods, and dulcifie with white Sugar a pound and a half. [Addition] Caraway seeds, Coriander Seeds, *ana.* seven drachms and a half, *Calamus Aromaticus*, *Zedoary*, *ana.* eleven drachms, fifteen Grains, Aniseeds, Cassia Lignea, *ana.* two ounces, three drachms, thirty Grains, Angelica Roots two ounces, three drachms, grains thirty, or Herb Angelica nine ounces, four drachms, grains thirty, white Sugar twelve ounces.

Worth. 'This is an excellent Cardiack, 'wonderfully strengthning the Heart, Stomach, and inward parts; 'tis a great Counter-poison and Preservative against the 'Plague, Measles, Small-pox, and other 'Pestilential and Infectious Diseases. The 'Dose is from half an ounce, to an ounce.

Aqua Absinthii, *or, Wormwood-Water.*

Composition the greater.

Distiller. Take of strong Proof Spirit sixteen gallons, Aniseeds bruised one pound, eight ounces, three drachms, grains twelve, Wormwood common, leaves and seeds stript and dry, three pound, six drachms, grains twenty four, Distill them into fine Goods, *S. A.* and dulcifie with white Sugar eight pound [Addition] Cinnamon, Cubebs, *ana.* ſix ounces, two ſcruples, grains eight; ſweet Fœnil-ſeeds, Aniſeeds, *ana.* twelve ounces, three drachms, grains ſix; Cloves, Caraway ſeeds, Nutmegs, *ana,* four ounces and a half, two drachms, grains ſix; Wormwood dry one pound, white Sugar, three pounds, twelve ounces.

Compoſition the leſſer.

Take of ſtrong Proof Spirit three gallons, Aniſeeds bruiſed four ounces, ſeven drachms, Wormwood common, leaves and ſeeds, ſtript and dry, ten ounces and a half, Diſtill them into fine Goods, and dulcifie with white Sugar one pound and a half. [Addition] Cinamon, Cubebs. *ana.* one ounce, one drachm, grains forty five, ſweet Fœnil ſeeds, Aniſeeds, *ana.* two ounces, three drachms, grains thirty, Cloves, Caraway ſeeds, Nutmegs, *ana.* ſeven drachms, grains thirty, Wormwood dry three ounces, white Sugar twelve ounces.

Beworth. ‘ This Water ſtops Vomiting, ‘ and provokes a good Appetite, it conſumes ‘ and expels Wind, and ſtrengthens the Sto- ‘ mach; wonderfully fortifying ſuch as are of ‘ a cold and moiſt Nature, and Conſtitution; ‘ it diverts Melancholy, and prevents many ‘ of thoſe Vapours, which otherwiſe would ‘ aſcend to the Head for its diſturbance; it ‘ eaſeth Gripes, and deſtroys Worms. The ‘ Doſe is the ſame with Aniſeed-Water.

Aqua

Aqua Meliſſæ, *or*, *Bawm-Water*:

Compoſition the greater.

Diſtiller: Take of ſtrong Proof Spirits ſixteen Gallons, Bawm dry four pound, twelve ounces, four drachms; Aniſeeds one pound, nine ounces, five drachms; Diſtill into fine Goods, and dulcifie with white Sugar eight pound: [**Addition**] Garden Thyme, Penny-royal; *ana.* five handfuls, Cardamums three ounces, grains thirty; ſweet Fœnil ſeeds, Aniſeeds, *ana.* twelve ounces, ſix drachms, grains thirty; Bawm dry one pound, nine ounces, four drachms; Nutmeg, Ginger, Calamus Aromaticus, Galingal, Cinamon, *ana.* ſix ounces, three drachms, grains fifteen.

Compoſition the leſſer.

Take of ſtrong Proof Spirit three gallons, Bawm dry thirteen ounces and a half, Aniſeeds four ounces, ſeven drachms; Diſtill into fine goods, and dulcifie with white Sugar a pound and a half. [**Addition**] Garden Thyme, Penny-royal, *ana.* a ſmall Pugil, Cardamums four ounces and a half, ſweet Fœnilſeeds, Aniſeeds, *ana.* two ounces, three drachms and a half; Bawm dry four ounces and a half; Nutmeg, Ginger, Calamus Aromaticus, Galingal, Cinamon, *ana.* one ounce, one drachm and a half, grains fifteen.

B-worth. ‘ This is highly eſteemed for
‘ Womens Diſeaſes, eſpecially in Hyſterick
‘ Paſſions, Vapours and Fits of the Mother;
‘ it ſhows its prevalency in comforting Wo-
‘ men in the Difficulty of Travail, not only
‘ ſtrengthning the Heart, whereby they are
‘ enabled the better to bear their pain, but
‘ alſo promoting a more quick and ſafe deli-
‘ very in which Caſe the Doſe may be one
‘ ounce or two.

Aqua Menthæ, *or, Mint-Water.*

Compoſition the greater.

Diſtiller. Take of high Proof Spirit ſix-teen gallons, Spearmint dry four pound, twelve ounces, two drachms, grains five, Aniſeeds beſt one pound, nine ounces, five drachms; and Diſtill into ſtrong Proof Spirits, and then dulciſie with white Sugar eight pound. [**Addition**] Spearmint dry, Aniſeeds, *ana.* one pound, twelve ounces, ſeven drachms, Calamus Aromaticus ſix ounces, three drachms, grains fifteen, white Sugar four Pound, four ounces.

Compoſition the leſſer.

Take of ſtrong Proof Spirit three gallons, Spearmint dry, four ounces, two drachms, grains five, Aniſeeds four ounces, ſeven drachms, diſtill into fine goods, and dulciſie with white Sugar one pound and a half.

[Ad-

[Addition] Spearmint dry, Aniſeeds, *ana.* four ounces, ſeven drachms; Calamus Aromaticus, one ounce, two drachms, one ſcruple, five grains, white Sugar twelve ounces.

P-worth. 'This Water is an excellent 'Cardiack, Splenetick and Stomachick, 'helping Concoction, and taking the 'Water off the Stomach; it prevents ſowre 'belchings, and hath a Specifick Virtue 'againſt Vomitings. The Doſe is from three 'drachms to ſeven or eight.

Aqua Roſmarini, *or, Roſemary Water.*

Compoſition the greater.

Diſtiller. Take of good Proof Spirit ſixteen gallons, Roſemary ſtript and dry, three pound, Aniſeeds, one pound, nine ounces, five drachms; Diſtill into fine goods, and then dulcifie with white Sugar, five pound. [Addition] Sweet Fœnil ſeeds, Cinnamon, *ana.* twelve ounces, ſix drachms and a half; Aniſeeds, Roſemary dry, *ana.* one pound, nine ounces, five drachms; Carrawayſeeds, three ounces, one drachm and a half, Spearmint dry, three handfuls, white Sugar four pound.

Com-

Composition the lesser.

Take of high Proof Spirit, three gallons, Rosemary stript and dry, nine ounces, Aniseeds four ounces, seven drachms; Distill into fine goods, and then dulcifie with white Sugar, half a pound. [Addition] Sweet Fennil seeds, Cinnamon, *ana.* two ounces, three drachms and a half; Aniseeds, Rosemary [illegible] *ana* four ounces, seven drachms; Ca[illegible] seeds, four drachms and a half; Spear[illegible], a competent quantity, white Sugar [illegible] ounces.

[illegible]worth. 'Rosemary water is an excel[illegible] Cephalick and Stomachick, for it comforts the Brain, revives the Senses, easing violent pains of the Head, it strengthens the Stomach, and is good against the Diarrhœa, Dysentery or *Irish* Flux, as also the Strangury, or difficulty of making Water: It may be safely Administred these three ways, *sc.* one ounce and a half to be drunk, given in a Clyster, or injected into the Yard.

Aqua Limoniarum aut Aurantiorum, *Limon, or, Orange Water.*

Composition the greater.

Distiller. Take of good Proof Spirits fixteen gallons, Limon or Orange Pills dry, three

three pound, Aniseeds the best one pound, nine ounces, five drachms, bruise the Pills and Seeds, and then distill into fine Spirit, and dulcifie with white Sugar eight pound. [Addition] Caraway seeds six ounces, four drachms, Aniseeds, Limon Pills dry, *ana.* one pound and a half, five drachms, grains six, white Sugar four pound: In the like manner and quantity you may make your Composition with Orange Pills dry.

Composition the lesser.

Take of good Proof Spirit three gallons, Limon or Orange pills dry, nine ounces, Aniseeds the best four ounces, eight drachms; bruise the pills and seeds, and then distill into fine Spirit, *Secundum Artem*, dulcifie with white Sugar one pound and a half. [Addition] Carawaysees one ounce, three drachms, grains fifteen; Aniseeds, Limon pills dry, *ana.* four ounces, seven drachms, white Sugar twelve ounces: In the like manner, and quantity you may make your Composition with Orange pills dry.

B-worth. ‘This is a great strengthener ‘of the spirits, Natural, Vital and Animal, ‘and by its fragrancy is very refreshing to ‘the Stomack, breaking away wind; 'tis also ‘a good Cordial restorative, opening Ob-‘structions, and being indued with a Balsa-‘mick Virtue, heals inward defects. The ‘Dose is from three drachms to six.

Aqua

Aqua Majoranæ, *or Marjoram Water.*

Composition the greater.

Distiller. Take of strong Proof Spirit sixteen gallons; sweet Marjoram dry, four pound, thirteen ounces; Aniseeds, one pound, nine ounces, five drachms; Caraway-seeds, six ounces, three drachms, grains fifteen; *Calamus Aromaticus* nine ounces, five drachms; bruise them, and distill into fine goods then dulcifie with white Sugar what is sufficient *Secundum Artem.* [**Addition**] Cinnamon eight ounces, Cloves three ounces, one drachm and a half; Limon pills dry four ounces, six drachms and a half, Sugar four pound.

Composition the lesser.

Take of strong Proof Spirit three gallons, sweet Marjoram dry, fifteen ounces; Aniseeds, four ounces, seven drachms; Caraway-seeds, one ounce, three drachms, grains five, Calamus Aromaticus, one ounce, seven drachms; bruise them and distill into fine good, *S. A.* and then dulcifie with white Sugar, one pound and a half. [**Addition**] Cinamon one ounce and a half; Cloves, four drachms and a half, Limon pills dry, seven drachms and a half, Sugar, twelve ounces.

A worth.

Physick. 'Tis good against the Infir-
'mities of the Liver and Spleen, and short-
'ness of Breath; 'tis a great Corroborator
'and strengthner of the inward parts. The
'Dose is from three drachms to six.

Aqua Meliphylli, *or, Balsamint Water.*

Composition the greater.

Distiller. Take of good Proof Spirit sixteen gallons, Balsamint dry, three pound, three ounces, one drachm and a half, Aniseeds best one pound and a half, one ounce, five drachms, Carrawayseeds six ounces, three drachms; Limon pills dry, twelve ounces, six drachms and a half; bruise them that are to be bruised, and then distill into strong Proof Spirit, and dulcifie with white Sugar eight pound, *S. A.* [Addition] sweet Fœnil, Cinnamon, *ana.* eight ounces, Nutmegs, four ounces, six drachms and a half, Sugar four pound.

Composition the lesser.

Take of good Proof Spirit three gallons, Balsamint dry, nine ounces, four drachms and a half; Aniseeds best four ounces, seven drachms, Carawayseeds one ounce, one drachm, Limon Pills dry, two ounces, three drachms and a half; bruise them that are to be bruised, and then distill into strong Proof pirits,

Spirits, and dulcifie with white Sugar, one pound and a half, *S. A.* [Addition] sweet Fœnil, Cinnamon, *ana.* one ounce and a half, Nutmegs seven drachms and a half, Sugar twelve ounces.

P-worth. 'This is a good Stomachick 'and Carminative. The Dose six or eight 'drachms.

Aqua Caryophyllorum, *or,* *Clove Water.*

Composition the greater.

Distiller. Take of high Proof Spirit sixteen gallons, Cloves one pound, Aniseeds one pound, nine ounces, five drachms, distill into fine goods, and then dulcifie with white Sugar, eight pound.

Composition the lesser.

Take of high Proof Spirit three gallons, Cloves three ounces, Aniseeds four ounces, seven drachms; distill into fine goods, and then dulcifie with white Sugar one pound and a half.

P-worth. 'This Water is esteemed very 'good for helping Digestion, breaking Wind, 'opening the Urinary passage and provoking 'Urine; for fortifying the Vital Spirits, and 'the Heart, the fountain thereof. The Dose 'is from two to four drachms.

Aqua

Aqua Cinnamomi Communis, *or, Cinnamon Water Common.*

Compoſition the greater.

Diſtiller. Take of ſtrong Proof Spirit ſixteen gallons, Cinnamon the beſt, eight pound, Aniſeeds, one pound; diſtill into fine goods, and then dulcifie with white Sugar twelve pound, *S. A.*

Compoſition the leſſer.

Take of ſtrong Proof Spirit three gallons; Cinnamon the beſt one pound and a half, Aniſeeds three ounces; diſtill into fine goods, and then dulcifie with white Sugar, two pound, four ounces.

Aqua Cinnamomi Propria, *or, Cinnamon Water Proper.*

Compoſition the greater.

Diſtiller. Take of good Proof Spirit ſixteen gallons, Cinnamon the beſt, and large, ſixteen pound; diſtill into fine goods: Then take white Sugar twenty pound, Roſewater ſix pound, ſix ounces, three drachms, make them into a Syrup, and dulcifie therewith, *S. A.* [**Addition**] Musk and Ambergreeſe, *ana.*

ana. two ſcruples, grains eight, white Sugar Candy inſtead of common white Sugar *qu. ſat. e. S. A.*

Compoſition the leſſer.

Take of good Proof Spirit three gallons, Cinnamon the beſt and large, three pound, diſtill into fine goods : Then take white Sugar, three pound, thirteen ounces, Roſewater one pound, three ounces, one drachm, make them into a Syrup, and dulcifie therewith, *S.A.* [Addition] Musk and Ambergreeſe, *ana.* grains nine, white Sugar Candy inſtead of common white Sugar, *qu. ſat. S. A.*

Obſerve, In reſpect that Musk for ſome cauſes may give offence to the Receiver; 'tis requiſite to omit the uſe thereof in ſome of your Water of this kind, to ſerve for ſuch particular uſes.

Aqua Cinnamomi Noſtra, *or, our Cinnamon Water.*

Worth. Take of our *Spiritus Vini Sulphurat* : one gallon (for when you make ſuch rich Cordial Waters, 'tis beſt to make uſe of ſuch Brandified Spirits as the Spirit of Malt, or any other bereaved of their ill Tang and Hogo, and then impregnated with an Azural Salt and Sulphur of a Vinous Nature) of the beſt Cinnamon in ſmall powder, one pound, four ounces, Sugar half a pound, Chryſtals of Tartar,

Tartar, four ounces; let them infuſe therein ten days, or the longer the better, and then diſtill into high Proof Spirits; and thus have you the true Spirit of Cinnamon, moſt proper for any Phyſical uſe whatever: But to allay it into a Cordial Water, you muſt proceed thus.

Take of freſh Cinnamon half a pound, ſpring Water three quarts, put them into your Alembick with its Refrigeratory, and diſtill over; and what Oyl comes will ſink to the bottom, the which you may ſeparate; and then to every quart of this Water add of Loaf Sugar one pound, and over a gentle warmth diſſolve it; and ſo with this you may allay your Spirit to Proof, or what height you pleaſe.

'Its Virtues are excellent againſt Vomit-'tings, weakneſs of the Stomach, and ſtink-'ing Breath; 'tis a good Cardiack, Pectoral, 'Lienick and Splenetick; comforting the 'Vital and Animal Spirits, giving ſtrength 'even to the Brain and Sinews. The Doſe 'is according as dilated, the weaker, one 'ounce, the ſtronger two or four drachms at 'the moſt.

Aqua Seminum Fœniculi dulc. *or, sweet Fœnil Seed Water.*

Composition the greater.

Distiller. Take of strong Proof Spirit sixteen gallons, sweet Fœnil seeds, eight pound, Carawayseeds six ounces, three drachms, Aniseeds one pound, nine ounces, five drachms; distil into fine goods, and then dulcifie with white Sugar eight pound. [**Addition**] Sweet Fœnil seeds eight pound, Caraway seeds six ounces, three drachms, grains fifteen, Aniseeds one pound, nine ounces, five drachms, Cinnamon twelve ounces, six drachms and a half, Cloves three ounces, one drachm and a half, Sugar four pound.

Composition the lesser.

Take of strong Proof Spirit three gallons, sweet Fœnil seeds one pound and a half, Carawayseeds one ounce, one drachm, Aniseeds four ounces, seven drachms; distil into fine goods, and then dulcifie with white Sugar one pound and a half. [**Addition**] Sweet Fœnil seeds one pound and a half, Carawayseeds one ounce, three drachms, grains five, Aniseeds four ounces, seven drachms, Cinnamon two ounces, three drachms and a half, Cloves four drachms and a half, Sugar twelve ounces

Pworth.

P-worth. *This Water takes off Stomachick Loathings, and creates an Appetite, ſtrengthening the Tones, imbibing ſharp humours, and expelling Wind. The Doſe is from half an ounce to an ounce and half.*

Aqua Calendularum, *or, Marigold Water.*

Compoſition the greater.

Diſtiller. Take of ſtrong Proof Spirit ſixteen gallons, Marigold Flowers new gather'd, pick'd clean, three pecks and a quarter; bruiſe them, ſweet Fœnil ſeeds, Aniſeeds, *ana.* one pound; diſtil into fine goods, and dulcifie with white Sugar eight pound. [Addition] Cinnamon, ſweet Fœnil, *ana.* half a pound, Caraway, Cloves, *ana.* three ounces, one drachm and a half, Marigolds three pecks, $\frac{1}{4}$, Sugar four pound.

Compoſition the leſſer.

Take of ſtrong Proof Spirit three gallons, Marigold Flowers, new gather'd, and pick'd clean, $\frac{3}{4}$ peck, or what more ſufficeth; bruiſe them; ſweet Fœnil ſeeds, Aniſeeds, *ana.* three ounces; diſtil into fine goods, and dulcifie with white Sugar, one pound and a half. [Addition] Cinnamon, ſweet Fœnil, *ana.* one ounce, four drachms, Caraway, Cloves, *ana.* four drachms and a half, Marigolds *q.s. e.* Sugar twelve ounces.

V-worth. *'Tis a wonderful strengthner, and as great a Preserver against any Infection whatsoever. The Dose is an ounce or two in the morning, especially when contagious Diseases do reign.*

Aqua Seminum Caruorum, *or, Caraway Water.*

Composition the greater.

Distiller. Take of high Proof Spirit sixteen gallons, Caraway seeds three pound, Aniseeds one pound, Rosemary dry six ounces, three drachms, Limon pills dry, Cloves, *ana.* four ounces, six drachms and a half, distil into fine goods, *S. A.* and dulcifie with white Sugar eight pound.

Composition the lesser.

Take of high Proof Spirit three gallons, Caraway seeds nine ounces, Aniseeds three ounces, Rosemary dry one ounce, one drachm; Limon pills dry, Cloves, *ana.* seven drachms and a half; distil into fine goods, *S. A.* and then dulcifie with white Sugar one pound and a half.

V-worth. *This Water hath been found very good for such as have been oppressed with cold and moist Stomachs, as also for such as have been subject to Wind in the Bowels, for it warms, comforts, and strengthens. The Dose is from three to six drachms.*

Aqua Nucum Moschatarum, *or, Nutmeg Water.*

Composition the greater.

Distiller. Take of strong Proof Spirit sixteen gallons, Nutmegs two pound, Aniseeds one pound, bruise them, and distil into fine goods, *S. A.* and then dulcifie with white Sugar, eight pound.

Composition the lesser.

Take of strong Proof Spirit three gallons, Nutmegs six ounces, Aniseeds three ounces, bruise them, and distil into fine goods, *S. A.* and then dulcifie with white Sugar one pound and a half.

Y-worth. *This Water cheers the Spirits, Natural, Vital, and Animal; it sweetens the Breath, and is a good Carminative and Diuretick. The Dose is the same with Caraway Water.*

Aqua Lavendulæ, *or*, *Lavender Water.*

Compofition the greater.

Diftiller. Take of high Proof Spirit fixteen gallons; Lavender Leaves dry, four pound, twelve ounces, fix drachms and a half; Lavender Flowers dry, three pound, three ounces, one drachm and a half; Mace, twelve ounces, fix drachms and a half; Nutmegs one pound, nine ounces, five drachms; Lavender Cotton dry, three pound, three ounces, one drachm and a half; Stæchados, twelve ounces, fix drachms and a half; bruife them that are to be bruifed, and diftil into Proof Spirit, *S. A.* dulcifie with white Sugar fixteen pound, or what lefs fufficeth.

Compofition the leffer.

Take of high Proof Spirit three gallons; Lavender Leaves dry, fourteen ounces, three drachms and a half, Lavender Flowers dry, nine ounces, four drachms and a half; Mace, two ounces, three drachms and a half; Nutmegs, four ounces, feven drachms; Lavender Cotton dry, nine ounces, four drachms and a half; Stæchados, two ounces, three drachms and a half; bruife them that are to be bruifed, and diftil into proof fpirit, *S. A.* dulcifie with white Sugar three pound.

Aqua

Aqua Lavendulæ Composita, *or, Lavender Water Compound.*

Distiller. Take Flowers of Lavender, Lilly of the Valley, *ana.* twenty four handfuls; piony, Tillia, Flowers of Rosemary, *ana.* half an handful, Sage, Cinnamon, Ginger, Cloves, Cubebs, Galingal, Calamus Aromaticus, Mace, Misseltoe of the Oak, *ana* one drachm and a half; piony roots, one ounce and a half; of the best Wine what sufficeth; infuse them in the Wine two days, and then distil in *Bal. Mariæ.*

V-worth. *'Tis good for such, as have Diseasy Ideas abounding, and are troubled with dulness of Spirit, as also against Falling-sickness, Convulsion Fits, and Infirmities of the Brain. The Dose is from one to three drachms.*

Observe, Here is no quantity of Spirits given, because the *Distillers* have a usual way in this thing to go by their own Experience, that is, they'll make them no richer of the Herbs, Seeds, and Spices, than as they'll answer their cost in the Sale; therefore they sometimes put two or three Cans more, than we prescribe; nay, and omit one half of the Ingredients, only observing, that according as the Water is called, to let that Herb, Seed, or Fruit, have the predominance of the Flavours; so that they go more by Custom than by Book; but for our part we don't in all things approve of this; for we love true prescriptions, tho'

 the

the Waters be something the dearer, and so to unite sound Theory and Practice together.

Aqua Salviæ, *or, Sage Water.*

Composition the greater.

Distiller. Take of strong Proof Spirit sixteen gallons; great Sage dry, four pound, twelve ounces, six drachms and a half; Red Sage dry, three pound, three ounces, one drachm and a half; Lavender Flowers, Sage Flowers, *ana.* one pound, nine ounces, five drachms; Lavender Cotton dry, Southernwood dry, *ana.* twelve ounces, six drachms and a half; Nutmegs one pound; bruise or beat them, as is most proper, and then distil into fine goods, *S. A.* and dulcifie with white Sugar sixteen pound, or what sufficeth.

Composition the lesser.

Take of strong Proof Spirit three gallons, great Sage dry, fourteen ounces, three drachms and a half, Red Sage dry, nine ounces, four drachms and a half, Lavender Flowers, Sage Flowers, *ana.* four ounces, five drachms, Lavender Cotton dry, Southern-wood dry, *ana.* two ounces, three drachms and a half; Nutmegs one ounce, bruise or beat them, as is most proper, and then Distil into fine goods, *S. A.* and dulcifie with white Sugar three pound. Aqua

Aqua Salviæ Composita, *or, Sage Water Compound.*

Distiller. Take Sage, Marjoram, Thyme, Lavender, Epithymum, Bettony, *ana.* one ounce; Cinnamon, half an ounce: Ireos, Roots of Cyprus, Calamus Aromaticus, *ana.* one ounce; Storax, Benjamin, *ana.* one drachm and a half; infuse them four days, in four pound of Spirit of Wine, and then distil in *Balneo.*

P-worth. *'Tis good for such as are cold and Phlegmatick, to revive the Spirits, and fortifie the digestive faculty, as also against oppressive Vapours, that disturb the Microcosm. The Dose is from two drachms to an ounce.*

Aqua Caryophillatorum, *or, Avens Water.*

Composition the greater.

Distiller. Take of good Proof Spirit, sixteen gallons; Avens Roots, six pound, six ounces, three drachms, grains five, Orrice Roots, Nutmegs, Yellow Sanders, Mace *ana.* three ounces, one drachm and a half; Lignum Rhodium, Saffron, Storax, Benjamin, *ana.* one ounce and a half, grains fifteen; Angelica Roots four ounces, six drachms and a half, Limon Pills Green, twelve ounces, six drachms

drachms and a half; sweet Fœnil seeds, Aniseed, *ana.* one pound, nine ounces, five drachms; Cloves, two ounces; Roman Wormwood, Mint dry, *ana.* four handfuls and a half; Red Roses, Stæchas Flowers, *ana.* six handfuls and a half; sweet Marjoram, Balm, Burnet, Thyme, all dry, *ana.* nine handfuls and a half; Alkermes Berries, three ounces, one drachm and a half; bruise them all that are to be bruised; and distil into Proof Spirit; *S. A.* and then dulcifie with Syrups thus made: Take Rosewater, six pound, six ounces, three drachms, grains fifteen; white Sugar sixteen pound; boyl it to a Syrup height, then strain it, and put it on the Fire again, adding thereto Confection of Alkermes, six ounces, three drachms and a half; Syrup of Gilly-Flowers, one pound, nine ounces, five drachms; Ambergreese (dissolved in Rosewater) four scruples, grains sixteen, let these boyl a little, till they be incorporated with the Syrup, and so keep it for use.

Composition the lesser.

Take of good Proof Spirit three gallons, Avens Roots, one pound, three ounces, one drachm, two scruples, grains five; Orrice Roots, Nutmeg, Yellow Sanders, Mace, *ana.* four drachms and a half; Lignum Rhodium, Saffron, Storax, Benjamin, *ana* two drachms, grains fifteen; Angelica Roots, seven drachms and a half; Limon pills green, two ounces, three drachms and a half; sweet

Fœnil-

Fœnilseeds, Aniseeds, *ana.* four ounces, six drachms; Cloves, three drachms; Roman Wormwood, Mint dry, *ana. q. s.* Red Roses, Stæchas Flowers, *ana. q. s. e.* sweet Majoram, Bawm, Burnet, Thyme, all dry, *ana. q. s. e.* Alkermes Berries, four drachms and a half; bruise them all that are to be bruised, and Distil into Proof Spirit, *S. A.* and then dulcifie with Syrups thus made: Take Rose water one pound, three ounces, one drachm, two scruples, grains fifteen; white Sugar, three pound; boyl it to a Syrup height, then strain it, and put it on the Fire again, adding thereunto Confection of Alkermes, one ounce, two drachms, one scruple, grains ten; Syrup of Gilliflowers, four ounces, seven drachms; Ambergreese (dissolved in Rosewater) grains eighteen, let these boil a little, till they be incorporated with the Syrup, and so keep it for use.

Y-worth. *This Water is a very great Cordial, Exhilarating the Spirits, strengthning and comforting all the inward parts; it not only preserves against the Consumption, but also strengthens and revives those that are in it. The Dose is from one to six scruples, according to the age and strength of the Patient.*

Rosa Solis.

Composition the greater.

Distiller. Take of strong Proof Spirit sixteen gallons; Cinnamon the best, twelve ounces, six drachms and a half; Cloves, three ounces, one drachm and a half; Nutmegs, Ginger, Carawayseeds, *ana.* six ounces, three drachms; Marigold Flowers, Aniseeds, *ana.* one pound, nine ounces, five drachms; bruise them, and Distil into strong Proof Spirit, *S. A.* Then add to the Distilled Water, Liquorice Spanish, one pound, nine ounces, five drachms, Raisins of the Sun, brown Sugar, *ana.* eight pound; Red Sanders, six ounces, three drachms; bruise the Liquorice, and Raisins, stir them well together, and let them stand twelve days, then being clear it may be drawn for use.

Composition the lesser.

Take of strong Proof Spirit three gallons, Cinnamon the best, two ounces, three drachms and a half, Cloves, four drachms and a half; Nutmegs, Ginger, Carawayseeds, *ana.* one ounce, one drachm; Marigolds, Aniseeds, *ana.* four ounces, seven drachms; bruise them, and Distil into strong Proof Spirit, *S. A.* Then add to the Distilled Water, Liquorice Spanish, four ounces, seven drachms;

Raisins

Raisins of the Sun, brown Sugar, *ana.* one pound and a half; Red Sanders, one ounce, one drachm; bruise the Liquorice and Raisins, stir them well together, and let them stand twelve days, then being clear it may be drawn for use. [**Addition**] Add to the Spirit half as much as the rule of every particular Ingredients therein expressed: And instead of Sanders, give it the Tincture of Roses, Gilliflowers, or Poppies, *S. A.*

Worth. *'Tis esteemed an excellent Water for strengthning the Stomach, expelling Wind, and fortifying the Sanguifying Faculty. The Dose is half an ounce.*

Ros Solis Proprius.

Composition the greater.

Distiller. Take of high Proof Spirit, sixteen gallons; Ros Solis gathered in due season, and clean picked, six pound, six ounces, three drachms, two scruples, grains five; Juniper Berries, four pound, twelve ounces, six drachms and a half; Sassafras rooted with the Bark; Carawayseeds, *ana.* six ounces, three drachms, two scruples, grains five; Marigold Flowers, one pound, nine ounces, five drachms; Aniseeds, two pound, six ounces, three drachms and a half; bruise them that are to be bruised, and Distil into fine Goods, *S. A.* Then take hereof ten pound, three ounces; add thereto of Aqua Pretiosa, dulci-

dulcified, one pound, nine ounces, five drachms; Liquorice bruised, one pound, nine ounces, five drachms; and then dulcifie with white Sugar, sixteen pound: If you add none of the aforesaid Water, then instead thereof, take Musk, one drachm and a half, grains six; Ambergreese, four drachms and a half, grains eight; colour it with the Tincture of Gilliflowers and Roses, what is sufficient, *S. A.*

Composition the lesser.

Take of high Proof Spirit three gallons, Ros Solis, gathered in due season, and clean pick'd, one pound, three ounces, one drachm, two scruples, grains five; Juniper Berries, fourteen ounces, three drachms and a half: Sassafras with the Bark; Carawayseeds, *ana.* nine drachms, two scruples, grains five; Marigold Flowers, four ounces, seven drachms; Aniseeds, seven ounces, two drachms and a half; bruise them that are to be bruised, and Distil into fine Goods, *S. A.* Then take hereof, one pound, twelve ounces, four drachms and a half; add thereunto of Aqua Pretiosa, four ounces, three drachms, dulcified; Liquorice bruised, four ounces, three drachms, dulcifie with white Sugar, what sufficeth: If you add none of the aforesaid Water, then take instead thereof Musk, grains eighteen; Ambergreese, grains twenty four; colour it with the Tincture of Roses, or Gilliflowers, what sufficeth, *S. A.*

V-worth. *This carries with it all the Virtues of the former; being alſo powerful in opening Obſtructions, relieving decayed Natures, and giving help in the Falling ſickneſs. The Doſe is from two to ſix drachms.*

Aqua Stomachica minor, *or, Stomach Water the leſſer.*

Compoſition the greater.

Diſtiller. Take of good Proof Spirit ſixteen gallons; Spearmints dry, Lovage Roots dry, Aniſeeds, *ana.* one pound, nine ounces, ſix drachms; Calamus Aromaticus, Ginger, ſweet Fœnil ſeeds, Imperatoria Roots, Wormwood dry and ſtript, *ana.* twelve ounces, ſeven drachms, two ſcruples; Caraway and Coriander ſeeds, *ana.* nine ounces, five drachms; Cummin ſeeds, Cloves, *ana.* four ounces, ſix drachms and a half; bruiſe them that are to be bruiſed; and then Diſtil into ſtrong Proof Spirit, *S. A.* and dulcifie with white Sugar, eight pound.

Compoſition the leſſer.

Take of good Proof Spirit three gallons, Spearmint dry, Lovage Roots dry, Aniſeeds *ana.* four ounces, ſeven drachms; Calamus Aromaticus, Ginger, ſweet Fœnil ſeeds, Imperatoria Roots, Wormwood dry and ſtript, *ana.* two ounces, five drachms, Caraway and

and Coriander ſeeds, *ana.* one ounce, ſeven drachms; Cummin ſeeds, Cloves, *ana.* ſeven drachms and a half; bruiſe them that are to be bruiſed; and then Diſtil into ſtrong Proof Spirit, *S. A.* and dulcifie with white Sugar one pound and a half.

Aqua Stomachica major, *or, Stomach Water the greater.*

Compoſition the greater.

Diſtiller. Take of ſtrong Proof Spirit ſixteen gallons; Calamus Aromaticus, nine ounces, five drachms; Guajacum green Bark, Avens Roots dry, Galingal, *ana.* ſix ounces and a half; Citron Pills dry, Orange pills dry, white Cinamon, *ana.* four ounces, ſeven drachms, grains fifteen; Wormwood common dry, Wormwood Roman dry, Spearmint, Roſemary tops, Coſtmary, ſweet Marjoram, wild Thyme, all dry, *ana.* three ounces, one drachm and a half; Nutmegs, Cinamon, *ana.* four ounces, four drachms, Cubebs, Cardamums, *ana.* two ounces, three drachms, grains fifteen; ſweet Fœnil ſeeds, Coriander ſeeds, *ana.* eight ounces; Aniſeeds two pound, ſix ounces, three drachms; bruiſe all that are to be bruiſed; and then Diſtil into ſtrong Proof Spirit, *S. A.* and dulcifie with white Sugar, ſixteen pound.

Com-

Composition the lesser.

Take of strong Proof Spirit three Gallons; Calamus Aromaticus one ounce, seven drachms; Guajacum green Bark, Avens Roots dry, Galingal, *ana.* twelve ounces; Citron Pills dry, Orange Pills dry, white Cinnamon, *ana.* one ounce, one drachm, two scruples, grains five; Wormwood common dry, Wormwood Roman dry, Spearmint, Rosemary tops, Costmary, sweet Marjoram, wild Thyme, all dry, *ana.* four drachms and a half; Nutmeg, Cinnamon, *ana.* six drachms; Cubebs, Cardamoms, *ana.* three drachms, two scruples, grains five; sweet Fœnil seeds, Coriander seeds, *ana.* one ounce and a half; Aniseeds, six ounces, one drachm; bruise those that are to be bruised; and then distil into strong proof Spirit, *S. A.* and dulcifie with white Sugar, three pound.

Aqua Stomachica nostra, *or, Our Stomach Water.*

B:worth. Take *Spirit. Vini Sulphurat.* mentioned in the Chapter of Rectification, ten Gallons, of Gascoigne Wine one Gallon, mix them together, and digest in the Still with a gentle warmth twenty four Hours, then add in of Ginger, Galingal, Nutmegs, Grains of Paradise, Cloves, *ana* four Ounces, Aniseeds, sweet Fœnil-seeds, Caraway-seeds, Hearts-

H ease,

case, *ana* eight Ounces, Sage, Mint, red Roses, the Flowers of the Lilly of the Valley, *ana* ten Ounces, Thyme, Pellitory Camomil, Lavender, Avens, *ana* four large Handfuls, Spanish Angelica Roots, Zedoary, Snake-root, *ana* five Ounces, Musk and Ambergreese, *ana* five Scruples, put on the Head, and lute all close, and let them remain with a gentle warmth twenty four Hours more, and then distil into high proof Spirit, *S. A.* To every Gallon of this add ten Ounces of our *Potestates Rosmarini*, and a Pound and a half of the Syrup of Rasberies, or Black Cherries, and let it refine, *S. A.*

Its Virtues. "'Tis a great Preservative 'against all pestilential and infectious Diseases, powerfully corroborating and strengthning the Stomach, being indued with such 'salutiferous Virtues, as that it will really 'perform as much as any other Stomachick 'whatever. The Dose is from two to four 'Drachms.

Usquebaugh.

Composition the greater.

Distiller. Take of strong proof Spirit sixteen Gallons, Aniseeds one Pound, nine Ounces, five Drachms, Cloves three Ounces, one Drachm and a half, Nutmegs, Ginger, Caraway-seeds, *ana* six Ounces three Drachms, distil into strong proof Spirit, *S. A.* then add

to

to the diſtilled Water Liquorice Spaniſh, Raiſins of the Sun, *ana* three Pound three Ounces, one Drachm and a half, bruiſe the Liquorice and Raiſins, and then dulcifie with brown Sugar eight Pound, ſtir them well together, and ſo let it ſtand ten days, and then (being fine) draw off, and keep it for uſe.

Compoſition the leſſer.

Take of ſtrong proof Spirit three Gallons, Aniſeeds four Ounces ſeven Drachms, Cloves four Drachms and a half, Nutmegs, Ginger, Caraway-ſeeds, *ana* one Ounce one Drachm, diſtil into ſtrong proof Spirit, *S. A.* then add to the diſtilled Water Liquorice Spaniſh, Raiſins of the Sun, *ana* nine Ounces four Drams and a half, bruiſe the Liquorice and Raiſins, and then dulcifie with brown Sugar one pound and a half, ſtir them well together, and ſo let it ſtand ten days, and (then being fine) draw it off and keep it for uſe.

Iriſh Uſquebaugh.

Exworth. Take of ſtrong Canary Wine a Quart, the beſt Tent one Pint, *Aqua Vitæ* one Gallon, put them into a Glaſs Veſſel, adding thereunto Raiſins of the Sun choice and ſtoned two Pound, Dates ſtoned, and the white Skin thereof pulled out, two Ounces, Cinnamon groſly poudered two Ounces, four good Nutmegs bruiſed, of the beſt Engliſh Liquorice ſliced and bruiſed one Ounce, ſtop the Veſſel

 very

very close, and let them infuse in a cold place six or eight days, then let the Liquor run through a Bag (called *Manica Hypocratis*) made of white Cotton.

Usquebaugh Royal.

R=Worth Take of *Aqua Vitæ Glauberis* three Gallons, Muskadine one Gallon, Raisins of the Sun stoned seven Pound, Figs one Pound and a half, Dates stoned, and the white skins pulled off, seven Ounces, Cinnamon eight Ounces, Nutmegs three Ounces, Cloves, broad Mace, *ana* one Ounce, English Liquorice twelve Ounces, let them infuse in a cold place for twenty days in a Vessel close stop't, and then let them run through an *Hypocrates Sleeve*, bottle it up carefully, adding thereunto of the Syrup of Quinces and Syrup of Limons *ana* four Ounces, of the well tinged Powers of Saffron two Ounces, let it refine it self, and keep it close stop't. [**Addition**] Powers of Musk and Ambergreese, Tincture of Pearl, *ana* drops twenty, so doth it become excellent and vitally fragrant.

'This is a most famous and excellent Liquor, 'fit indeed for such as its Name and Superio-'rity belongs unto; it is a most estimable Jew-'el for such as are inclined to Melancholy, to 'drink now and then a quarter of a Spoonful 'thereof, 'tis so great a Stomachick, that it 'helps the digestive Faculties, prevalent in 'Surfeits, and the defects of the Lungs, as 'Phthisick, Consumption, causing Expectora-

'tion;

'tion; in brief, 'tis equal to any Cordial Spi-'rit whatever for fortifying the Natural, Vi-'tal and Animal Spirits. The Dose is from 'two to six Spoonfuls at the most.

Aqua Bezoartica, *or, Bezoar Water.*

Prescription the first, Composition the greater.

Distiller. Take of the Leaves and Roots of Celandine twenty one Handfuls, Rue six Handfuls, Scordium twelve Handfuls, Dittany of Creet, Carduus Benedictus, *ana* nine Handfuls, the Roots of Zedoary, Angelica, *ana* two Ounces two Drams, the inward Pill of Citron and Limon, *ana* three Ounces six Drams, Clovegilliflowers eight Ounces four Drams, red Roses, Centaury Flowers the least, *ana* one Ounce four Drams, let those be bruised that are to be bruised, and cut that are to be cut, and put them into the proper Vessel, and pour on them of the best Spirit of Wine and Malaga Wine *ana* ten Quarts one Pint, let them all steep three days, adding Vinegar of Cloves and Juice of Limons *ana* six Pound, and let them be distilled in *Balneo* in a large Glass Cucurbit with its proper Helm and Recipient. [**Addition**] Cinnamon two Ounces two Drams, Cloves one Ounce seven Drams, Venice Treacle two Ounces two Drams, Camphir four Drams, Troches of Vipers three Ounces, Mace one Ounce and a half, the Wood of Aloes six Drams, Yellow Saunders one Ounce one Dram, the Seeds of Carduus Benedictus six Ounces, the Kernels of Citrons two Ounces two Drams; the *Modus* of its Preparation is either to digest these with the former, and distil them over together at once, or else after the first part is distilled to add to the Liquor this Addition, and distil a second time in *B. M* with a most gentle Fire, and after you have removed a third of the Aereal Spirit, you may cohobate the rest two or three times to get the Virtue of the Ingredients out; your Liquors you may add together, and let it refine according to Art.

Composition the lesser.

Take of the Leaves of the great Celandine, together with the Roots thereof, three Handfuls and a half, Rue two Handfuls, Scordium four Handfuls, Dittany of Creet, Carduus, *ana* an Handful and half, Roots of Zedoary and Angelica, *ana* three Drams, the outward Rind of Citrons and Limons, *ana* six Drams, the Flower of Wall Gilliflowers one Ounce and a half, red Roses, the lesser Centaury, *ana* two Drams, Cloves, Cinnamon, *ana* three Drams, *Andromachus*'s Treacle three Ounces, Mithridate an Ounce and half, Camphir two Scruples, Troches of Vipers two Ounces, Mace two Drams, Lignum Aloes half an Ounce, Yellow Saunders one Dram and a half, the Seeds of Carduus one Ounce, the Seeds of Citron six Drams, cut those things that are to be cut, and let them be macerated

three

three days *in Spiritus Vini Glauberis*, and Muskadine, *ana* three Pints and a half, Vinegar of Wall Gilliflowers, and the Juice of Limons, *ana* a Pint, let them be distilled in the Glass Vessel before described in *B*. Observe, that after something more than one half of the Liquor is distilled off from either of these two Compositions, then the remainder in the Vessel must be strained through a linnen Cloath, and gently evaporated to the thickness of Honey, which is called the *Bezoar Extract*.

N. worth. We think it convenient to hang in the Neck of the Alembick Pearl prepared, white Amber, *ana* three Ounces, Oriental Bezoar and Ambergreese *ana* six Scruples, and when the Preparation is over what remains may be added to the Extract, then do both Spirit and Extract obtain a Nature something agreeable to the Name, and doubtless the Virtues are more powerful, *being an excellent Sudorifick, Alexipharmick, and Antifebritick, and prevalent against all pestilential and infectious Diseases; 'tis not in vain said of it, that it resists Melancholly, and chears the Spirits, comforting such as are in a languishing Nature, or Consumptive.* The Dose is from one Dram to an Ounce in Scordium or Honey-suckle-water, first in Mornings and last at Nights, but for such as are afflicted with Fits let them take it in the time of the Paroxism.

Aqua Mathiæ, *or, Doctor Mathias his VVater.*

Composition the greater.

Distiller. Take of Lavender Flowers three Gallons, pour on them of the best Spirit of Wine ten or twelve Gallons, the Vessel being closely stopped let them macerate in a gentle heat, or in the Sun for the space of seven days, and then distil in an Alembick with its Refrigeratory, and you have a Spirit of Lavender, to which add Sage, Rosemary, Betony, *ana* three Handfuls, Borage, Bugloss, Lillies of the Valley, Cowslips, *ana* six Handfuls, let the Flowers be fresh and seasonably gathered, and macerated in a Gallon of the best Spirit of Wine, or rather *Spiritus Vini Glauberis*, and mix it with the aforesaid Spirit, adding thereunto the Leaves of Bawm, Motherwort, Orange-Tree, newly gathered, the Flowers of Stæchados, Oranges, Bayberries, of each three Ounces, and after they are digested three days let them be distilled again, to which add of the outward Rind of Citron, and the Seeds of Peony, *ana* two Ounces two Drams, Cinnamon, Nutmegs, Mace, Cardamoms, Cubebs, Yellow Sanders, Lignum Aloes, of each one Ounce and a half, the best Jujubes, the Kernels taken out, one Pound and a half, let them digest twenty one days, then strain the Liquor from the Drugs, to to which add prepared Pearl six Ounces, prepared Emrald one Dram, Ambergreese, Musk, Saffron, red Roses, Sanders, *ana* three Ounces, Yellow Sanders, Rinds of Citrons dried, *ana* three Drams, let all these Species be tied in a silken Bag and hang'd in the foresaid Spirit.

Composition the lesser.

Take of Lavender Flowers one Gallon, Spirit of Wine three Gallons, prepare it as before directed, then take the Flowers of Sage, Rosemary, Betony, of each a Handful, Borage Bugloss, Lilly of the Valley, Cowslips, of each two Handfuls, the Flowers, being truly gathered, and macerated in a Gallon of the *Spiritus Vini Glauberis*, must be added to the Spirit of Lavender, as the former, together with the Leaves of Bawm, Motherwort, Orange-Tree, newly gathered, the Flowers of Stæchados, Oranges, Bayberries, of each an Ounce, and so digest and distil, as before directed, then add the outward Rinds of Citron six Drams, the Seeds of Peony husked six Drams, Cinnamon, Nutmegs, Mace, Cardamoms, Cubebs, Yellow Saunders, of each half an Ounce, Lignum Aloes one Dram, the best Jujubes, the Kernels taken out, half a Pound, digest and prepare as the former; to which Liquor add of prepared Pearl two Drams, prepared Emrald one Scruple, Ambergreese, Musk, Saffron, red Roses, Sanders, of each an Ounce, Yellow Sanders, Rinds of

Citrons

Citrons dried, of each a drachm; let these Spices be tyed in a Silken bag and hanged in the foresaid Spirit. [Addition.] The Essence of Musk and Ambergreese, *ana.* Drops twenty, the Mel of Black-cherries, and of Rasberries, *ana.* five ounces, the Syrup of Quinces, two ounces, so let it refine *S. A.*

Be-worth. *This is a most excellent Cordial, wonderfully strengthning the principal faculties, good in Epilepsies, Convulsions, Palsies and all Diseases of the Nerves; 'tis also excellent good to wash the wound bitten by any Venemous Creature, or to bath any grieved part; the Dose inwardly, is from one drachm to three, either* per se, *or in Wine.*

Aqua Scorbutica, *or,* French's *Scorbutick Water.*

Composition the greater.

Distiller. Take of the Leaves of Garden and Sea Scurvey-grass, picked and cleansed, of each eighteen pound, let them be bruised and the Juice pressed forth, to which add the Juice of Brook-lime, Water-cresses, of each one pound and a half, of the best White-wine, three gallons, thirty six whole Limons cut, of the fresh Roots of Briony, twelve pound, of the fresh Roots of Horse-Raddish, six pound, of Winter's bark one pound and a half, of Nutmegs, twelve ounces, let them

them be macerated three days and then Distilled.

Composition the lesser.

Take of the Leaves of Garden and Sea Scurvey-grass, picked and cleansed, of each six pounds, let these be bruised and the Juice pressed forth; to which add of the Juice of Brook-lime, Water-cresses, of each half a pound, of the best White-wine eight Pints, twelve Limons cut, of the fresh Roots of Briony four pound, the fresh Roots of Horse-Raddish two pound, of Winter's bark half a pound, Nutmegs four ounces; let them be macerated three days, then Distill: [Addition.] Syrup of Mustard two ounces, Syrup of Elder three ounces, Tincture of Coral and Milk of Pearl, of each Drops forty, mix them *S. A.*

Usworth. *This is a most excellent Anti scorbutick, not only good in the Scurvy, but also prevalent in the Jaundice and other refractory Diseases. The Dose is from half an ounce to two ounces, first in a Morning and last at Night.*

Aqua Aperitiva, *or, a Carminative opening Water.*

Composition the greater.

Distiller. Take Roots of Eringo, Vipers-Grass, Fern, the greater Centaury, of each one ounce and a half, Roots of Fœnil, Barks of of Capparis, Tamarisk, Ash, of each one ounce, one drachm, Barks of Citrons, seven drachms and a half, seeds of Carduus Benedictus, Cichorie, of each one ounce and a half, seeds of Endive, Cresses, Citrons, Scariol, of each six drachms, Polytricon, Adianthum, Ceterach, Dodder, Scolopendria, Bettony, Endive, of each four handfuls and an half; tops of Thyme, Epithymum, Hops, Flowers of St. John's Wort, Broom, Borage, Bawm, of each three handfuls, small Raisins, three ounces, Cinnamon four drachms and a half; *Spec. Dialacc.* one drachm and a half, Water of Carduus Benedictus, Hops, Scolopendria, Paul's Bettony, of each three pound, Rhenish-wine, seven pound and a half; let them stand two days in a warm place, in a Vessel close stopp'd, afterward Distill them in *Balneo.*

Composition the lesser.

Take Roots of Eringo, Vipers-Grass, Fern, the greater Centaury, of each half an ounce, Roots of Fœnil, Barks of Capparis, Tamarisk, Ash, of each three drachms, Bark of Citrons two drachms and a half, seeds of Carduus Benedictus, Cichory, of each half an ounce; seeds of Endive, Cresses, Citrons, Scariol, of each two drachms, Polytricon, Adianthum, Ceterach, Dodder, Scholopendria, Bettony, Endive, of each a handful and a half; tops of Thyme, Epithymum, Hops, Flowers of St. Johns Wort, Broom, Borrage, Bawm, of each one handful; small Rasins, one ounce, Cina-

Cinamon, one drachm and a half; *Spec. Dialacc.* half a drachm; Water of Carduus Benedictus, of Hops, of Scolopendria, of *Paul's* Bettony, *ana.* one pound, Rhenish Wine, two pound and a half; let them stand two days in a warm place, in a Vessel close stopp'd, afterward Distill them in *Balneo.* [Addition] *Aqua Vitæ Glauberis*, two pound; the Juice of Goose-berries, two pound, or in place thereof Goose-berry Wine, made as prescribed in our *Brit. Magazine of Liquors*; the Juice of Black-berries, half a pound, the Juice of Buckthorn Berries, six ounces, Cinnamon and Nutmegs, *ana.* two ounces, Sugar half a pound; let it be prepared *Secundum Artem.*

P-worth. *'Tis a prevalent Water to open the Obstructions of the whole Body, especially of the Liver, Spleen and Mesentery: the Dose is from two drachms, to six or eight, two or three times a day.*

Aqua Vulneraria, or *VVound VVater.*

Composition the greater.

Distiller. Take Plantain, Rib-wort, Bone-wort, Wild Angelica, Red Mints, Bettony, Agrimony, Sanicle, Blew-Bottles, White-Bottles, Scabius, Dandelion, Avens, Honey-Suckle Leaves, Bramble buds, Haw-thorn buds and Leaves, Mugwort, Daisie Roots, Leaves and Flowers, Wormwood, Southern-wood, of each four handfuls; boyl all these in two gallons of White-wine, and as much Spring Water till one half be wasted; and when it is thus boyled, strain it from the Herbs, and put to it two pound of Honey, and let it boyl a little after; then divide this into two parts, the one part head with common ferment, and let it ferment for three days, then add into every Quart thereof, a pound of *Aqua Vitæ Glauberis*, and Distill into high Proof Spirits. *S. A* [Addition] Cinnamon, Lignum Aloes, of each four ounces, Mirrh, Aloes and Saffron, of each one ounce, then perfume and colour, as in other precious Waters, and dulcifie with Syrup of Cinnamon and Syrup of Poppies, of each three ounces; and lastly, add in of *Laudanum Liquidum*, four drachms, Tincture of Coral six drachms; let it refine *S. A.*

Worth. *'Tis not only excellent for such as are wounded, but also for those that are subject to internal bleedings; it mortifies the Corrosive, Acid, and Saline juices, so sweetens and thickens the Blood; the Dose in such a case is, from half an ounce, to one ounce and half, according to the Age, Strength and Constitution of the Patient, every three hours; as also every two hours, for three days together, for such as are subject to Vomiting of Blood. The first Water made by decoction is very famous in curing Wounds, Imposthumes and Ulcers, such cures have been done by it that few may credit it; it first gives ease in a very short time, and then performs the cure, if not so far declined, as that the highest Specificks, will not prevail: For inward wounds you must*

take

take this with the other; but this Morning and Evenings, four or five spoonfuls at a time, and that all times of the day. If the Wound be outward it must be washed therewith, and Linen Cloaths wet in the same be applyed thereto. Note that the Herbs herein contained must be gathered in their true Signature, as also in the Month of May.

Aqua Mariæ, *or, the Ladies Water.*

Composition the greater.

Distiller. Take Sugar Candy, four pound, Canary Wine, one pound and half; Rose-water, one pound, boyl them well into a Syrup to which add *Aqua Cælestis*, eight pound, Ambergreese, Musk, *ana.* one drachm, grains twelve; Saffron one drachm, Tincture of Coral (saith Dr. *Boylwharfe*) one ounce, Yellew Sanders infused in *Aqua Cælestis*, hereafter described, one ounce; Distil or make a clear Water, *S. A.*

Composition the lesser.

Take Sugar Candy one pound, Canary Wine six ounces, Rose-water four ounces, make of these a Syrup, and boyl it well, to which add of *Aqua Imperialis*, two Pints, Ambergreese, Musk, of each eighteen grains, Saffron fifteen grains; Yellow Sanders infused in *Aqua Imperialis*, two drachms; [**Addition**] *Aqua Preciosa*, hereafter expressed, half an ounce

ounce, the Tincture of Coral, Bezoar, and the aurified Sulphur of Antimony, *ana.* two drachms, refine and unite, *S A.*

Vertues. *'Tis very good against the Plague, and all Pestilential Diseases, and an excellent Counterpoison; it strengthens the Spirits, and is prevalent against fainting and swooning fits; it is good against most cold Diseases of the Head, Brain and Stomach, and principally for Men, but not so good for Women, unless the Musk and Ambergreese be left out. The Dose is a spoonful or two, first in the Morning, and last at Night going to Bed.*

Aqua Anticolica Nostra, *or, Our Water against the Colick.*

Composition the greater.

Vertues. Take of Daucus, or wild Carrots, twelve ounces, Aniseeds, eight ounces, Cumminseeds, three ounces, two drachms, Cinnamon four ounces and a half; Mace, Cloves, Nutmegs, *ana.* seven drachms, Galingal one ounce and half; Calamus Aromaticus dried, two ounces and a half, the dried Rind of Oranges and Limons, *ana.* six ounces, Galls and Grains, *ana.* one ounce, two drachms; infuse these by way of Fermentation, for twelve days in the fragrant Wine of Camomile Flowers five Gallons; Elder-wine a gallon and half; then pour on five Gallons of Proof Spirit, and draw into high

high Proof, or fine goods; dulcifie with white Sugar four pound. [Addition] Apricocks, Centaury, Agrimony, Adonis, of each half a pound; Palma Christi, Hart-wort, Lavender of each six ounces; Yarrow and Zedoary, of each four ounces, white Sugar four pound, *Tinctura Anadyna*, or *Laudanum Liquidum*, four ounces, refine *S. A.*

Composition the lesser.

Take of Daucus, or wild Carrots, four ounces, Aniseeds, two ounces, five drachms, one scruple, Comminseeds one ounce, two scruples; Cinnamon one ounce and a half; Mace, Cloves, Nutmegs, *ana.* two drachms, one scruple; Gallingal half an ounce; Calamus Aromaticus dried, seven drachms the dried Rind of Oranges and Limons, *ana.* two ounces, Galls and Grains, *ana.* three drachms, one scruple; infuse these by way of fermentation for twelve days, in fragrant Wine of Camomile Flowers, one gallon and a half, Elder-Wine half a gallon, then pour on a gallon and half of Proof Spirit; and draw into high Proof or fine goods, dulcifie with white Sugar, one pound, four ounces, [Addition] Apricocks, Centaury, Agrimony, Adonis, of each two ounces, five drachms, Palma Christi, Heart-wort, Lavender, of each two ounces, Yarrow and Zedoary, of each one ounce, two drachms, grains fifteen, white Sugar one pound, six ounces, *Tinctura Anodyna*, or *Laudanum Liquidum*,

quidum, one ounce, two drachms, two ſcruples, refine, *S. A.*

Its Vertues. *It is not only good againſt the Cholick, but alſo oppreſſion of Wind in the Stomach and Bowels, how offenſive ſoever it be, and the more eſpecially if you dilate it in a little cold diſtilled Water of Yarrow, and ſweeten it with the Syrup of Poppies, and drink it as a Cordial, in which Caſe you may take half a Pint at two Draughts, with an Hours intermiſſion; 'tis moſt excellent alſo for the Gripes in ſucking Children, being taken to the quantity of a Spoonful or Spoonful and half in Breaſt Milk.*

Aqua noſtra in Vermes, *or, Our Worm-Water.*

Compoſition the greater.

R-worth. Take of Hellebore, Savin, Broom Flowers and Tops, *ana* a Peck, pour thereon the Water of Tanſie, Rue and Peach Flowers, *ana* two Gallons, adding thereunto Sugar five Pound, and with the common Ferment let them ferment five or ſix days, then take of Wormſeed bruiſed one Pound, Wormwood Tops and Seeds ſix Handfuls, Peach Flowers three Handfuls, the fine Shavings of Hartſhorn a Pound, ſtrong proof Spirit ten Gallons, diſtil into fine Goods, and dulcifie with White Sugar eight Pound. [**Addition**] Agrimony, Cedar, Elecampane, Garlick, Muſtard, Nettles, Hartſtongue Leaves, *ana* an Handful,

Aloes

Aloes bruised six Ounces, Chrystals of Tartar half a Pound, fine Sugar six Pound.

Composition the lesser.

Take of Hellebore, Savin, Broom Tops and Flowers, *ana* a quarter of a Peck, pour thereon of the Water of Tansie, Rue and Peach Flowers, *ana* four Pints, adding thereunto Sugar one Pound four Ounces, and ferment with the common Ferment five or six days, then take of Wormseed bruised four Ounces, Wormwood Tops and Seeds two Handfuls, Peach Flowers a large Pugil, the fine shavings of Hartshorn four Ounces, strong proof Spirit two Gallons and a half, distil into fine Goods, and dulcifie with White Sugar two Pound. [**Addition**] Agrimony, Cedar Elecampane, Garlick, Mustard, Nettles, Hartstongue Leaves, *ana* half a Pugil, or a small Pugil, Aloes bruised one Ounce and a half, Chrystals of Tartar four Ounces, fine Sugar one Pound and a half.

Its Virtues. *'Tis prevalent against all kinds of Worms both in Young and Old, for being dilated into a Cordial with the Syrup of the three first Herbs it becomes a Medicine not to be surpassed by any thing short of a Specifick. The Dose is from half an Ounce to an Ounce, according to the Age, Nature and Condition of the diseased: you must observe to take it seven Mornings together fasting.*

Aqua nostra Convulsiva, *or, Our Water against the Convulsion.*

Composition the greater.

R-worth Take of Black Cherries bruised with their Kernels two Gallons, of the Flowers of Lavender nine Handfuls, White Mustard Seeds bruised three Ounces, mix them together and put some Ferment to them, and let them ferment for five or six days, then add two Gallons of our sulphurated Spirit of Wine, or rather *Aqua Vitæ Glauberis*, and distil into fine Spirits according to Art.

Then take of *Ros Vitrioli*, (which is the Water that distils from Vitriol in the Calcination thereof) six Quarts, Misseltoe of the Oak and Peony, *ana* two Ounces two Drams, of Rue three Handfuls, Juniper Berries three Ounces, Bay berries an Ounce and a half, Camphir an Ounce, Rhubarb sliced two Ounces and a half, Cats Blood two Pound, Spirit of Turpentine three Ounces, digest ten days, and then distil in *Balneo Mariæ*; you may mix this with the former in equal parts. [Addition] Bawm, Deanwort, Capers, Coffee, Hearts-ease, Mastich, Brightwort, St. John's Wort, Spiknard, Rosemary and Valerian, *ana* six Handfuls, fine Sugar eight Pound.

Composition the lesser.

Take of Black Cherries bruised with their Kernels four Pints, of the Flowers of Lavender

der two Handfuls and a half, White Mustard-seed bruised six Drams, mix them together, and put some Ferment to them, and let them ferment for five or six days, then add of our sulphurated Spirit of Wine, or rather *Aqua Vitæ Glauberis*, four Pints, and distil into fine Spirits, *S A*.

Then take of *Ros Vitrioli* three Pints, Misseltoe of the Oak, Peony, *ana* four Drams one Scruple, Grains ten, Rue one Handful and a half, Juniper-berries half an Ounce two Drams, Bay-berries three Drams, Camphir two Drams, Rhubarb sliced five Drams, Cats Blood half a Pound, Spirit of Turpentine six Drams, digest ten days, and then distil in *Balneo Mariæ*; you may mix this with the former in equal parts. [**Addition**] Bawm, Dean-wort, Capers, Coffee, Hearts-ease, Mastich, Brightwort, St. *John*'s Wort, Spikenard, Rosemary, Valerian, *ana* one Handful and a half, fine Sugar two Pound.

Its Virtues *'Tis excellent for the weakness of the Head, not only good against Convulsions, but also for Vertigo's, and most Diseases of the superior Region; it strengthens the Sinews, and expels Wind out of the Head and Stomach, giving powerful relief in Hypochondriack and Hysterick Passions, 'tis a prevalent help for Children that have Convulsive Fits, and especially if given in a few drops of our* **Essentia Crani-humani**, *spoken of in our* **Chymic Rational** *The Dose is from a Dram to two, and from thence to an Ounce, or an Ounce and half, according to the Age and Strength of the Patient.*

Thus (Reader) I have given the *Basis* and Foundation of such Waters as hitherto have not been so plainly published, that so they may be of some Advantage to such as languish under the Burthen of Diseases for want of their precious Virtue, for whose Benefit we shall yet proceed as follows, first of

Aqua pretiosa, *or*, *Precious Water.*

Composition the greater.

Distiller. Take of strong proof Spirit sixteen Gallons, of the Roots of *Enula Campana*, Avens, Angellica, Cyprus, *Calamus Aromaticus*, Sassafras, *ana* eight Ounces, Zedoary, Galingal, *ana* six Ounces three Drams, Cassia Lignea, Lignum Rhodium, Yellow Sanders, *ana* four Ounces six drams and a half, the dry Peels of Citrons and Oranges, *ana* nine ounces four drams, Cinnamon white, Nutmegs, Mace, Ginger, *ana* eight ounces, the choicest Cinnamon two Pound, Cloves, Cardamoms, Cubebs, *ana* three Ounces six Drams, sweet Chervil Seeds, Basil Seeds, *ana* five Ounces three Drams, Coriander Seeds, sweet Fennil-seeds, *ana* one Pound, Aniseeds two Pound, bruise them and distil into proof Spirits, and then dulcifie with white Sugar twenty four Pound, *S. A.* and let it stand till it be fine, then draw it off, and add Musk one Dram two Scruples, Ambergreese six Drams two Scruples, then let it clear, and draw it off for use.

Com-

Compoſition the leſſer.

Take of ſtrong proof Spirit three Gallons, Roots of *Enula Campana*, Avens, Angelica, Cypreſs, *Calamus Aromaticus*, Saſſafras, of each one Ounce and a half, Zedoary, Galingal, *ana* one Ounce, one Dram, Caſſia Lignea, Lignum Rhodium, yellow Sanders, *ana* ſix Drams and a half, the dry peels of Citron and Orange, *ana* one ounce ſix drams grains fifteen, Cinnamon white, Nutmegs, Mace, Ginger, *ana* one ounce and a half, Cinnamon beſt ſix ounces, Cloves, Cardamoms, Cubebs, *ana* ſix drams, ſweet Chervil Seeds, Baſil Seeds, *ana* one ounce one dram, Coriander Seeds, ſweet Fœnil Seeds, *ana* three ounces, Aniſeeds ſix drams, bruiſe them and diſtil into ſtrong proof Spirit, and then dulcifie with fine white Sugar four Pound and a half, *S. A.* let it ſtand till it be fine, then draw it off, and add Musk grains eighteen, Ambergreeſe one dram grains twelve, then let it clear and draw it for uſe.

The Syrup for dulcifying the Water is thus to be made.

Take Apricocks, Quinces, Cherries, *Engliſh* Currans, of each what ſufficeth, all full ripe, and of equal weight, when they are thus prepared as followeth.

Prepare the Quinces and Apricocks, take out the Stones and Kernels and ſlice them ve-ly thin, stone the Cherries, and bruise them and the Currants; then lay them in a flat bason or pan thus: A lane of Fruit of a fingers thickness, and then a lane of white powder Sugar of like thickness, and so proceed in order, lane upon lane, till all be laid into the bason; then pour on good *Aqua Vitæ*, gently, till all be covered therewith, and so let it stand two hours, then bruise, or posh them all together, and press out the Juice as dry as possibly you can through a thick linnen bag; then take the Juice, and let it stand till it be settled clear, which Juice, by a gentle Exhalation in a hot bath, boyl up to a Syrup height, according to Art, and keep it for use, To every eight pound of the Spirit, put a pound of this Syrup, and when [illegible] draw it off for use.

[illegible] *'Tis a rare and excellent Water* [illegible] *are inclined to Melancholy; for it* [illegible] *the Heart, revives the Spirits, pre-* [illegible] *comforting the Sences, and will de-* [illegible] *in the time of Contagious Diseases,* [illegible] *Plagues and malignant Feavers.* The *Dose* is from two *Drachms* to an *Ounce*.

Aqua Carminativa, or Wind-water.

Composition the Greater.

Distiller Take of strong proof Spirit 16 Gallons, Enula Campana roots dry, Aniseeds, of each one pound nine ounces and five drams, Cyprus roots, bark of the roots of

Bay-

Bay-tree, or as much leaves, Sassafras with the bark, Cinnamon white, of each nine ounces, four drams, two scruples, and five grains, Calamus-aromaticus, Orange pills dry, of each six ounces and three drams, Clary, red Mint, Calamint, Elder-flowers, Camomile-flowers, of each eight ounces, sweet Fennel-seeds, Carraway-seeds, Angelica-seeds, of each six ounces and three drams, Coriander-seeds, Cardamums, Cubebs, Grains of Paradise, Cloves, and Ginger, of each four ounces, Pepper long and white of each two ounces, bruise them all grosely, and distil into fine Goods *S. A.* and then dulcifie with white Sugar sixteen pound, and draw it off for use when it is perfectly clear.

Composition the Lesser.

Take of strong Proof Spirit three gallons, Ennula campana-roots dry, Aniseeds, of each four ounces and seven drams, Cyprus-roots, bark of the roots of Bay-tree, or as much leaves, Sassafras with the bark, Cinamon white, of each one ounce, six drams, and fifteen grains, Calamus-aromaticus, Orange-pills dry, one ounce and a dram, Clary, red Mints, Calamint, Elder-flowers, Camomile-flowers, of each an ounce and an half, Sweet-Fennel-seeds, Caraway-seeds, Algelica-seeds, of each one ounce and a dram, Coriander-seeds, Cardamums, Cubebs, Grains of Paradise, Cloves, and Ginger, of each six

ſix drams, Pepper long and white, of each three ounces, bruiſe them all groſely, and diſtil into fine goods *S. A.* then dulcifie with white Sugar three pound, and draw it for uſe when it is perfectly clear.

Aqua Sudorifica, *or* Water to procure Sweat.

Compoſition the greater.

Diſtiller. Take of ſtrong Proof Spirit 16 gallons, Butter-bur-roots dry, three pound, three ounces, one dram and an half, Valerian (common) roots, Aniſeeds, of each one pound and an half, one ounce, and five drams, Vincetoxicum-roots, Saſſafras-roots with the bark, of each twelve ounces, ſix drams and an half, Angelica herb dry, Carduus Benedictus, Great-Valerian herb and roots, all dry, Scordium, of each, one pound, three ounces, one dram and an half, Cowſlip-flowers, Marigold-flowers, of each, one pound, Juniper-berries, two pound, bruiſe them all, and diſtill into fine goods *S. A.* and then dulcifie with white Sugar ſixteen pound.

Compoſition the leſſer.

Take of Strong Proof Spirit three gallons, Butter-bur-roots dry, nine ounces, four drams and an half, Valerian (common) roots, Aniſeeds, of each four ounces ſeven drams, Vin-

Vincetoxicum-roots, Sassafras-roots with the bark, of each two ounces, four drams, and an half, Angelica herb dry, Carduus Benedictus, Great-Valerian herb and roots all dry, Scordium, of each, three ounces, four drams and an half, Cowslip-flowers, and Marigold-flowers, of each three ounces, Juniper-berries, six ounces, bruise them all, and distil into fine goods, S. A. and then dulcifie with White Sugar three pound.

Vertue. *This Water is very excellent in provoking Sweat, the Patient drinking an Ounce thereof, and then to be covered close in bed; by which means many Disseasy Idea's will be dissipated and carried off, and the Spirits and Body strengthened*

Aqua contra Crapulam, or Surfeit Water.

Composition the greater.

Distiller. Take of strong Proof Spirit sixteen gallons, Juniper-berries, three pound, three ounces, one dram and an half, Enula Campana roots dry, one pound, nine ounces, and five drams, Calamus aromaticus, Galingale, of each six ounces, and three drams, Wormwood, Spearmint, and Red-Mint all dry, of each four ounces, Caraway-seeds, Angelica-seeds of each three ounces, one dram and an half, Sassafras-roots with the bark, and White Cinamon, of each four ounces, six drams and an half, Nutmegs, Mace, Cloves, and Ginger, of each, one ounce

ounce and an half, two ſcruples, and five grains; Red-Poppy-flowers, ſix pound, ſix ounces and an half, Aniſeeds four pound, bruiſe them all, and diſtill into fine goods *S. A.* and then dulcifie with white Sugar ſixteen pound.

Compoſition the leſſer.

Take of ſtrong Proof Spirit three gallons, Juniper-berries nine ounces, four drams and an half, Ennula Campana roots dry four ounces and ſix drams, Calamus-aromaticus, and Galingale, of each an ounce and a dram, Wormwood, Spearmint, and Red-Mint all dry, of each ſix drams, Carraway-ſeeds and Angelica-ſeeds, of each four ounces and a half, Saſſafras-roots with the bark, white Cinamon, of each ſeven drams and an half, Nutmegs, Mace, Ginger, and Cloves of each two drams and fifteen grains, Red-Poppy-flowers one pound three ounces and an half, Aniſeeds, twelve ounces, bruiſe them all, and diſtil into fine goods, *S. A.* and dulcifie with white Sugar three pound.

V-worth. *This Water is not only good for Surfeits, but alſo for Feavers, Agues, and Obſtructions, and all others, wherein a ſharp and Acid ferment too much affects the Blood. The Doſe is from half an ounce to an ounce. If in this Doſe you mix two or three drams of our* **Spiritus Mundus**, *and drink it two or three times a day, it will cure moſt Pleuriſies without Vena-ſection.*

Aqua

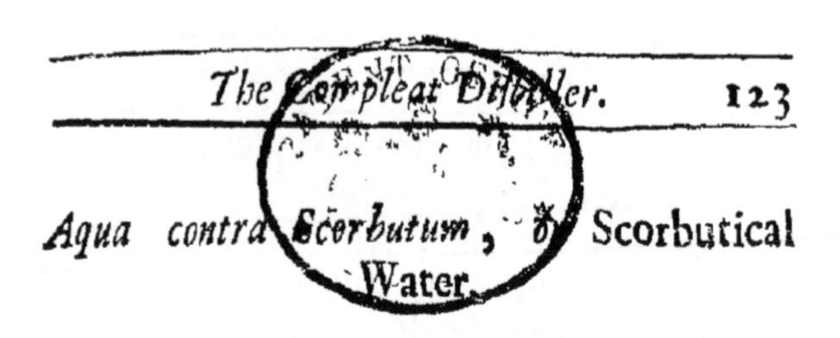

Aqua contra Scorbutum, or Scorbutical Water.

Compoſition the Greater.

Diſtiller. Take of ſtrong Proof Spirit, ſixteen gallons, Horſe-radiſh-roots dry three pound three ounces one dram and an half, Enula-Campana-roots dry, Aniſeeds, of each one pound nine ounces and five drams, Water-creſſes, Winter-creſſes and Garden-creſſes, Taragon, Balſamint, Scurvy-graſs (garden) Wormwood, Brook-lime, Trefoile (water) Sweet-Chervile, of each nine ounces and an half two ſcruples and five grains Arſmart twelve ounces ſix drams and an half, Muſtard, Bank-creſs, Rocket, Radiſh, of the ſeeds of each, four ounces ſix drams and an half, Citron-pils, Orange-pils dry, Cinamon white, and Mace, of each ſix ounces three drams and fifteen grains, bruiſe them all, and then diſtil into fine goods *S. A.* and dulcific with white Sugar ſixteen pound or what ſufficeth. For uſe take ſeven parts of this Spirit, and one part of the Juice of Limmons (or more) mingle them together, and dulciſie with white Sugar what ſufficeth.

Compoſition the leſſer.

Take of ſtrong Proof Spirits three gallons Horſe-reddiſh-roots dry nine ounces four drams

drams and an half, Enula-Campana-roots dry, and Aniseeds of each four ounces and six drams, Water-cresses, Winter-cresses, Garden-cresses, Taragon, Balsamint, Scurvy-grass (garden) Wormwood, Brook-lime, Trepoile (water) and Sweet-Chervile of each one ounce six drams and five grains, Arsmart two ounces three drams and an half, Mustard, Bank-cress, Rocket, Radish, of the seeds of each seven ounces and an half, Citron-pils, Orange-pils dry, Cinamon white, and Mace, of each one ounce one dram two scruples and five grains, bruise them all and then distil into fine goods *S. A.* and dulcifie with white Sugar three pound: For use take seven parts of this Spirit, and oné part of Juice of Limmons (or more) mingle them together and dulcifie with white Sugar, what sufficeth.

Virtues. *This Water is excellent for purifying the Blood and for carrying off the Scorbutick Acidity, by way of mortification; for it sweetens the same all one, as Spirit of Wine doth the Spirit of Salt; The Dose for such is from two to six drams, twice or thrice a day.*

Aqua contra Pestilentiam, or Plague-Water.

Composition the Greater.

Distiller. Take of strong Proof Spirit sixteen gallons, Butter-bur-roots dry one pound nine ounces and five drams, garden and

and common Valerian-roots both dry, Angelica-roots, Imperatoria, Gentian, Enula-Campana, Snake-grafs-roots of each nine ounces and an half two fcruples and five grains, Contrayerva, Zedoary, and Galingale, of each fix ounces three drams and fifteen grains, Rue-leaves dry, white Horehound, Scordium, Carduus-Benedictus of each eight ounces, Elder-flowers, Lavender, and Mace of each four ounces, fix drams and an half, Citron-pils dry, Juniper-berries of each twelve ounces fix drams and an half, Green Walnuts with the husks one pound nine ounces and five drams, Venice Treacle, and Mithridate, of each three ounces one dram and an half, Anifeeds (beft) two pound fix ounces three drams and an half, Camphire an ounce and an half two fcruples and five grains; Diftil into fine goods *S. A.* and dulcifie with white Sugar fixteen pound.

Compofition the leffer.

Take of ftrong Proof Spirit three gallons, Butter-bur-roots dry four ounces and feven drams, Garden and Common Valerian-roots, both dry, Angelica-roots, Imperatoria, Gentian, Enula-Campana, Snake-grafs roots, of each one ounce and an half two drams and five grains, Contrayerva, Zedoary, and Galingale, of each one ounce one dram two fcruples and five grains, Rue-leaves dry, White-Horehound, Scordium, Carduus Benedictus, of each one ounce and an half, Elder-der-flowers, Lavender and Mace, of each ſeven drams and an half, Citron-pils dry, Juniper-berries of each two ounces three drams and an half Green Walnuts with the husks, four ounces aud ſeven drams, Venice Treacle, and Mithridate, of each four drams and an half, Aniſeeds beſt ſeven ounces two drams and an half, Camphire two drams and fifteen grains; diſtil into fine Spirit *S. A.* and dulcifie with white Sugar three pound.

For Uſe, let the party infected take of this Water one Ounce mingled with warm Poſſet-drink (or any other Water proper in that caſe) and be kept warm, and ſweat well thereon.

Aqua noſtra contra Peſtilentiam, *or* our Plague-Water.

Y-worth. Take of Spaniſh Angelica Roots half a pound, Engliſh Angelica-leaves, Rue, and Sage, of each three handfuls, Long-Pepper, Nutmegs, and Ginger of each one ounce and an half, *Venice* Treacle and Mithridate of each four ounces, *Malaga* Wine two quarts, *Aqua Vitæ Glauberis* one gallon, digeſt twenty days, and then diſtil into fine Spirit *S. A.* [Addition] Contrayerva, *Virginia* Snake root, and Zedoary of each three ounces, the Powers of Vipers four ounces, Camphire one ounce, Syrup of Wine Vinegar one pound, with which refine down after diſtilled.

This

This Water is an incomparable preservative in, and against, the Plague, Small-Pox, Measles, and all Pestilential and Contagious Diseases; Two Spoonfuls being taken three or four times a day as a Cordial: 'Tis good also for all cold Stomacks, want of Digestion and the like.

Aqua Florum, or Water of Flowers.

Composition the greater.

Distiller. Take of strong Proof Spirit sixteen gallons, and put it into a wide-mouth'd-pot (or other Vessel) stop'd very close; take these several Flowers following, in their Seasons, and being clean pickt, put them to the Spirit in the Pot, *viz.* Cowslips, Woodbine, Stock-Gilli-flower of all the three sorts, Damask-Roses, Musk-Roses, Sweet-Briar-flowers, Lillium Convallium, Jesemin, Citron-flowers, Orange-flowers or their pils dry, Tillia-flowers, Garden-Limmon and wild Thyme-flowers, Lavender, Marigold, Chamomile, Mellilot, and Elder-flowers, of each twelve ounces six drams and an half; being furnished with all your Flowers, as above, when you would distil them, add thereunto Aniseeds three pound three ounces one dram and an half, Coriander-seeds one pound nine ounces and five drams, bruise the seeds, 'twere also best to bruise all the Flowers, as you put them up into the Spirit, for the more orderly working, Distil into fine Spirit S. A then add to the distill'd Water Roses, Gilliflowers and Elder Flowers, of each one pound nine ounces and five drams; after twelve days Infusion it may be drawn off, then dulcifie it with white Sugar sixteen pound, and being fine it may be drawn for use.

Composition the lesser.

Take of strong proof Spirit three gallons, put it into a wide mouth'd Pot (or other Vessel) stopt very close, take these several Flowers following in their seasons, and being clean pickt put them to the Spirit in the Pot, *viz.* Cowslips, Woodbine, Stock-gilliflower of the three sorts, Damask-Roses, Musk-Roses, Sweet-brier Flowers, Clovegilliflowers, Lillium Convallium, Jesemin, Citron and Orange Flowers, or their pills dry, Tillia-flowers, Garden-Limmon and Wild Thyme-flowers, Lavender, Marigold, Chamomile, Mellilot, Elder Flowers, of each two ounces three drams and an half; being furnished with all your Flowers as above, when you would distil them add thereunto Aniseeds nine ounces four drams and an half, Coriander Seeds four ounces and seven drams, bruise the Seeds, and 'twere also best to bruise all the Flowers as you put them up into the Spirit, for their more orderly working; distil into fine Spirit S. A. then add to the distilled Water Roses, Gilliflowers, Elder Flowers, of each four ounces and seven drams, after twelve days Infusion

it

it may be drawn off, then dulcifie it with white Sugar three pound, and being fine it may be drawn for uſe.

P-worth. *This is a great Cordial for ſtrengthening and refreſhing the Spirits, and therefore proper for thoſe who are troubled with Hypochondriack Melancholy. The Doſe is from one Dram to five, according to the Age, Strength and Condition of the Patient.*

Aqua Frugum, *or Water of Fruits.*

Compoſition the greater.

Diſtiller. Take of ſtrong proof Spirit ſixteen gallons, Juniper-berries ſix pound ſix ounces three drams and fifteen grains, Quince and Pippin parings both dry of each three pound three ounces one dram and an half, Limmon-pills, Orange-pills dry, of each one pound nine ounces and five drams, Nutmegs ſix ounces three drams and fifteen grains, Aniſeeds three pound three ounces one dram and an half, Cloves three ounces one dram and an half, diſtil into fine Spirit *S. A.* to the Spirit add Strawberries, Raſberries bruiſed, of each eight pound, ſtir them well together, and after ten days, it being clear, may be drawn off, then dulcifie with Syrup made as is taught in *Aven*'s Water, and ſo let it ſtand till clear, and then draw it off for uſe.

Composition the lesser.

Take of strong Proof Spirit three gallons, Juniper-berries one pound three ounces one dram two scruples and five grains, Quince and Pippin parings both dry of each nine ounces four drams and a half Limmon-pills, Orange-pills dry, of each four ounces and seven drams, Nutmegs one ounce one dram two scruples and five grains, Aniseeds nine ounces four drams and an half, distil into fine Spirit *S. A.* to the Spirit add Strawberries, Rasberries bruised, of each one pound and an half, stir them well together, and after ten days, it being clear, may be drawn off, then dulcifie with Syrup made as is taught in *Aven*'s Water, and so let it stand till it be clear, and then draw it off for use.

P-worth. *This is a great Carminative, expelling Wind, good in Surfeits and Fevers, it abates Thirst. The Dose is from one Dram to five in some proper Vehicle, or dilated to a Julep.*

We having thus run through the Prescriptions of such which are varied into a greater and lesser Composition, we shall add some Observations, and then proceed to lay down some particular Waters that are purely for the use of such as would supply the Defect of an Apothecary when not near, &c.

You are first to observe, that in the distilling of these Waters you must not make use of the Wooll in the Head, for that will be apt to suck and drink in too much of the oleous part,

part, and ſo conſiderably deſtroy the Virtues of the Waters and altho' there will often come over a white thick ſhadowary Oil towards the latter end, by which the pure fine Spirits are troubled and made thick, yet we ſay that this may be thus prevented: Take a fine *Holland* Cloth and rub one ſide of it very well with Black Lead, and bind the ſide ſo rubb'd inwardly towards the end of the Worm, and this will keep the thickneſs back, as Experience demonſtrates.

But as to rich and coſtly Waters, you need not draw ſo long, and yet no Loſs, for what remains being fermented will give a very good Spirit for other beginnings; and altho' in every Receipt the way to colour, perfume and dulcifie the ſame is ſhewed, yet the *Diſtiller* as ſeldom regards it as he doth the quantity of Spirits to the *Pondus* of Herbs and Spices, for they are led by that Rule which will return moſt Profit into their Pockets; their general way is thus, they make a Syrup with ordinary Sugar, and too too often Treacle, having firſt decocted Braſil, Sanders, or the like, to colour the ſame, and then ſtrain the whole thro' a Canopy, and ſo add it to the Water to allay and dulcifie; one of their Preſcriptions is thus,

For Red Water.

Take of Spring-water one Gallon, or rather of the purified Liquor for Allays, of red Sanders one pound, Braſil half a pound, decoct these in the Water closely stopt on the Embers so long until you obtain all the Tincture from the Wood, then the Wood is strained out, to which quantity of Water you add six or eight pound of Treacle, or course Sugar, and let it gently simper, then clarifie with the Whites of ten or twelve Eggs, and strain it through a fustian Canopy; this you add to twenty or thirty Gallons of common *Aqua Vitæ*, more or less, according as it is in strength, and you would have it in sweetness; then to fine it 'tis usual to take Flour and the Whites of two or three Eggs, and with a spoonful or two of Yeast you beat them well together, adding thereunto a scruple of Musk, and ten grains of Ambergreese, and put them in a small Bag, the which you let hang by the Bunghole into your Liquor, and in fourteen days it will be fit for Sale. Now these following Simples are generally made use of for colouring your Liquors withal, *viz. Reds*, with *Rose Leaves*, *Poppy Leaves*, *Clovegilliflowers*, *Turnsole*, *Root Alkanet*, *Cochenele*, *Juices*, *Cherries*, *Rasberries*, *Mulberries and Backberries*. For Yellows, *Saffron*, *Turmerick and Yellow Sanders*. But seeing we must colour this way, we think it convenient to add our Opinion concerning the same, which is; if you use Woods, whether Brasil, Sanders, *&c.* that you decoct them in the cold distill'd Water of the Herb, appropriated to the Water, or else in cold distill'd Rose-water, twenty four Hours on gentle Embers, and then strain forth, and add of fine clean Sugar, boil up

and

and clarifie with a sufficient quantity of Whites of Eggs, and so let it pass through the Canopy or Fustian Sleeve, and then add it to the Waters you intend to dulcifie; and as for the Perfumes you add in, it is best that they be ground very well in a Mortar with some of the Spirits, and then added, or else let them be dissolved in it (close luted) in a gentle heat, and then added to the quantity, otherwise your Waters will want that smell to perfume them which only radical Dissolution obtains. Now for tender Leaves, as Poppies, Roses, *&c.* you had best also to take out their Tinctures, by some of the Spirit in a Vessel (close luted) in *Balneo*, which you must repeat so often till they remain pale, the which you must add to your quantity with your Sweets, and that you fine it with, let your Fruits and Berries be separated from their Stones, and strained so as that they may not be broken therein, for then it will make the pleasant Juice bitter; to these so prepared you may add your Sugar, and proceed as hath been directed *S. A.* by such Variations as Experience must prompt you in; thus have we laid down what is sufficient for any reasonable and industrious Person to build his Practice on, so that what remains is only to give you the Prescriptions of those rich and costly Waters promised.

Aqua mirabilis.

Take Cloves, Cubebs, Galingal Mace, Nutmegs, Cardamums, and Ginger, of each two Drams, the Juice of Salendine one Pint, Spirit of Wine two Pints, White Wine six Pints, infuse all these twenty four Hours, and then distill off four Pints by an Alembick.

B-worth. *This is of admirable force and virtue to preserve the Body from the Apoplexy, and all Diseases of the Nerves, it is very good against the Palsie, Convulsion and Cramp, as also for cold Stomachs. The Dose is from two Drams to half an Ounce.*

Aqua mirabilis nostra.

B-worth. Take Cloves, Galingal, Cubebs, Mace, Cardamums, Nutmegs and Ginger, of each three Drams, Bawm, Sage, Betony, Bugloss and Cowslip Flowers, all gathered in their prime, of each one Handful, the Juice of Salendine one Pint and an half, *Aqua Vitæ Glauberis* three Pints, the Wine of black Currans two Gallons, digest twenty four Hours, and distil off one Gallon in *Balneo Mariæ.*

This hath all the Virtues of the former in Superiority, more Cordial, thence wonderfully strengthening the Heart, Stomach, and principal Vessels, and therefore by us often called **Aqua Corobo-rans.** *The Dose is the same with the former.*

Dr. Stephens's *Water.*

Take of Gascoign Wine two Gallons, Ginger, Galingal, Cinnamon, Nutmegs, Grains, Aniseeds, Fennel-seeds, and Caraway-seeds, of of each two Drams, Sage, red Mints, red Roses, Thyme, Pellitory, Rosemary, Wild Thyme, Camomile, and Lavender, of each two Handfuls, beat the Spices small and bruise the Herbs, letting them macerate twelve Hours, stirring them now and then, distil by an Alembick or Copper Still with its Refrigeratory, keep the first Quart by it self, and the second by it self. *N. B.* that the first Quart will be the hotter, but the second the stronger of the Ingredients.

Virtues. *It is very excellent in strengthening the Heart, fortifying the Spirits, relieving languishing Nature. The Dose is from one Dram to two.*

Aqua Imperialis.

Take of the Rind of Citrons and Oranges dried, Nutmegs, Cloves, and Cinnamon, of each four Ounces, the Roots of Flower-de-luce, Cyprus, Calamus Aromaticus, Zedoary, Galingal, and Ginger, of each one Pound, of the tops of Lavender and Rosemary, of each four Handfuls, the Leaves of the Bay Tree, Marjoram, Bawm, Mints, Sage, Thyme; the Flowers of White and Damask Roses, of each one Handful, Rose-Water eight Pints, the best White Wine two Gallons, bruise what must be bruised, then infuse them all twenty four Hours, after which distil.

Virtues. *This Water strengthens and corroborates the Heart, and is therefore Good for such as are subject unto faintings, swoonings, and Pal-*

pitations

pitations of the Heart, and is a preservative against Apoplexies, the Dose is from one dram to three.

Aqua Cælestis.

Take of Cinamon, Cloves, Nutmegs, Ginger, Zedoary, Galingale, Long Pepper, Citron pill, Spicknark, Lignum Aloes, Cubebs, Cardamums, Calamus Aromaticus, Mace, Ground-pine, Germander, Hermodactyls, Tormentil, White Frankincense, the pi h of Dwarf Elder, Juniper-berries, Bay berries, the Seeds and Flowers of Motherwort, the Seeds of Smallage, Fennel and Anise, the Leaves of Sorrel, Sage, Felwort, Rosemary, Marjoram, Mints, Penny-Royal, Stechados, the Flowers of Elder, Red and White Roses, of the Leaves of Scabious, Rue, the lesser Moonwort, Egrimony, Centaury, Fumitary, Pimpernal, Sowthistle, Eyebright, Maidenhair, Endive, Red Saunders, Aloes, of each four ounces, pure Amber, the best Rhubarb, of each four drams, dried Figs, Raisins of the Sun, Dates stoned, sweet Almonds, Grains of the Pine, of each two ounces, of the best *Aqua Vitæ* to the quantity of them all, of the best hard Sugar two pound, of white Honey one pound; then add the Root of Gentian, Flowers of Rosemary, Pepperwort, the Root of Bryony, Sowbread, Wormwood, of each an ounce. Now before these are distill'd, quench Gold being made Red hot oftentimes in the aforesaid Water; put therein

therein Oriental Pearls, beaten ſmall two pound, and then diſtil it after twenty four hours Infuſion.

Y-worth. *This is a very good Cordial Water, prevailing againſt Malignant and Peſtilential Feavers, and a great reſtorative to ſuch as are in Conſumption, it comforts the Heart, and revives drooping Spirits; 'tis very hot in Operation; you muſt not exceed half a dram for the largeſt Doſe without the Advice of a Phyſitian; in Feavors mix it with cooling Juleps.*

Aqua Noſtra Multifera Virtutum, or our Water of Many Virtues.

Y-worth. Take Bawme, Sage, Bettony, Bugloſſe, Cowſlips, all gather'd in their prime, of each a handful, Motherwort, Bay-Leaves, of each a handful and half, Mary-gold-flowers two handfuls, flowers of Roſemary, Lavender, Lillies of the Valley, Roſa-ſolis, of each four handfuls, the Juice of Salendine two pound, Saffron two ounces, Lignum Aloes an ounce and half, Turmerick four ounces, Spirit of Wine ſix Quarts, digeſt all ſix days, and then diſtil in *B. S. A.*

This Water is excellent in the Diſeaſes of the Head, Breaſt and Heart, Liver and principal parts, fortifying the Faculties, and ſtrengthning Nature, as far as can be expected from ſimple Cordial Spirits without being enriched with ſome Mineral Sulphurs, the which will be ſhown in our Spagyrick Philoſophy Aſſerted, and

Spa-

Spagyrick Philosophy's Tryumph. Now by the way obſerve, that moſt of theſe Waters or Spirits, are too ſtrong to be taken alone, Nature not loving to ride in fiery Chariots, 'tis beſt therefore that they be dilated and reduced into Cordials, the way by which tis performed, will be ſhown in our **Medicina rationalis.**

Crollii Aqua Theriacalis Camphorat. Or *Crollius* his Treacle Water Camphorated.

Take of Andromachus his Treacle ten ounces, the beſt Myrrh five ounces, the beſt Saffron one ounce, Camphire four drams, mix them together, then pour upon them of the beſt Spirit of Wine twenty ounces, and let them ſtand twenty four hours in a warm place, then diſtil them in Balneo with a gradual Fire; Cohobate the Spirit three times.

V-worth. *This Water is of Excellent Virtue againſt the Peſtilence, and other Feavers; 'tis a very good Counter-Poyſon and good for thoſe that have been bit by any Venemous Creature, or ſuch as have the French Pox; for it drives forth all virulent Humours from the Heart, and is a great Cordial. The Doſe is from half an ounce to an ounce.*

Aqua

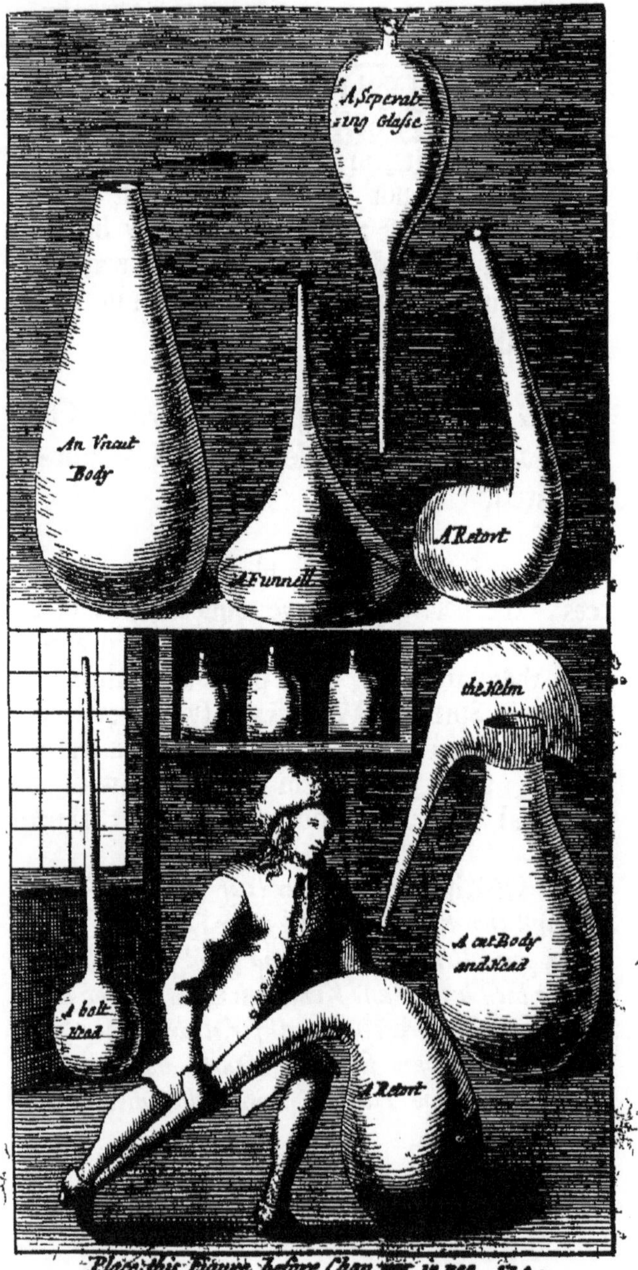

Place this Figure before Chap [illegible] *in pag.* 139.

Aqua Composita contra Scorbutum, or a Scorbutical Water.

Take of the Leaves of both sorts of Scurvey Grass, being made very clean, of each twelve pound; let these be bruised, and the Juice pressed forth; to which add the Juice of Brooklime, Juice of Water Cresses, of each a pound, of the best white Wine sixteen Pints, twelve Lemmons cut, of the fresh Roots of Bryony eight pound, of the fresh Roots of Horse-Radish four pound, of the Bark of Winteran one pound, of Nutmegs eight ounces; let them macerate three days, and then distil *S. A.*

Vertue. *This Water is Excellent for the Scurvy, with all the Symptoms that attend the same, 'twill radically cure those that are not too Rebellious in a Month or six Weeks time, if you take two Spoonfuls thereof in a Morning and Evening.*

I could indeed inlarge my self with various other Prescriptions, but I think it needless, seeing you have here what is sufficient to accomplish any *Distiller*; nay paradventure more than ever you may have occasion to make, so that others of a more Superior and Higher Order will be superfluous; as to such as have a desire to know more, thinking them necessary in their Medicinal practice, let them resort to our *Medicina Rationalis*, where

where they shall find them under the head of such Diseases as they are appropriated to: And for those that would be curious and have variety of chargeable Prescriptions, let them apply themselves to the *London Dispensatory*, and other Authors wherein they are prescribed: But as to such as desire the healing Virtues of one single Cordial which hath been found for many years to supply the place of many others, such we advise to our *Spiritus Prophylacticus Imperialis*, treated of in our *Spagyrick Phylosophy asserted*; for this indeed is various ways to be ordered, and that to such an advantage, as that it answers all that can be desired from any thing of this Nature; and therefore for the good of such as languish under deplorable Diseases we thought it requisite to give its Virtue and Use: First of the Spirit, and then of the way of dilating it into a Cordial.

Spiri-

Spiritus Prophylacticus Imperialis, or *the Antipeleptick Powers, Soveraign for all the Diseases of the Head, Womb-Fits, sudden surprisals, and infectious Diseases, being a general Cordial for all Diseases incident to the Body.*

As to its Preparation, 'tis given in our *Spagyrick Philosophy Asserted.*

Its Virtues in General.

This is a great Cordial, truly helping Nature, inwardly or outwardly applyed, and is of admirable benefit to poor fainty drooping Spirits and weak Nature, and a great Reliever and Comforter of Old Aged people, Strengthning and Comforting the Heart and Stomach, prevalent against Wind, Chollick, Gripes, Yellow-Jaundice Cough and Colds, and such like Distempers: And also Bruises and Contusions, wither'd and benumbed Members and Cramp; 'tis efficatious against Cold, moist Diseases of the Head, Stomach and Heart; as Apoplexies, Falling Sickness, Palsies, Trembling, Head-ach, Megrim, Vertigo Carus, Lethargy, Sleepiness and Dimness of Sight, cold Rheums, Catarrhs, Rhumatisms, Old Aches of the Back and Loyns, stinking breath; as also good against Convulsions.

Its Use and Dose.

For any Bruise, Squatt, Aches, or weak and decayed parts, you must dip a Cloth therein, and lay it four or five times double on the part, and at last having repeated this three or four times bind it fast thereon: For the Diseases of the Face and Head, you must annoint your Face and Temples, and take the savours up your Nostrils; For Rickets in Children, it must be applyed as well outwardly as inwardly, chafing the grieved part with the clear Spirit before the Fire; Dipping a Scarlet cloath in it, and laying it on the part affected, repeating it as often as occasion requires, and swathing from the Arm-pits to the Groins with a Linnen Swath: For weak and pained Limbs the same Method is to be observed as before.

'Tis also an Excellent preserver for dead Bodies; for if you wash the dead over with it two or three times, and then strike over all the Body with our double **Spiritus Odontugiasus**, *it preserves the same a considerable while, without being embowell'd; and more especially if you afterward apply to the Mouth, Stomach, Navel, and bottom of the Belly some of our* **Elixir Proprietatis Helmontii** *with a Spunge, by which method the Dead shall be not only preserved, but also kept from giving the least Annoyance or Evil Smell to any that shall come a near it; or the least infection, although they died of an infectious Disease; for if you repeat the use of these three or four times, the*

poy-

poyſonous Venom will be totally mortified. Now of what moment might this be in preſerving people in the Family, for the Chambers are kept ſweet, and the Perſon, if never ſo groſs, from purging, as experience manifeſts. Thus having given you its External uſes, we ſhall now proceed to the Internal ones, *Viz.* as it is dilated into a Cordial.

Cordialis Noſtra Generalis; or our General Cordial.

Take *Spiritus Prophelacticus Imperialis*, well tinged with *Pilula Nepenthe noſtr.* one pound, the fragrant Wine of Camomile Flowers, Yarrow and Daucus two pound, *Mel Vegetabile qu. ſa. e.* to Dulcifie it into a Cordial; to which add of the Radical Tincture of Gold, Bezoar, and the Milk of Crabs Eyes, of each Gutt. 20. ſhake them well together, then let it ſtand and ſettle, and decant the clear, ſo is it prepared.

This Cordial is in many Caſes as profitable unto the Sick, as their Food, eſpecially for weakneſs, Faintneſs, and violent Illneſs, that ſeize on people, for this will (if deſign'd for Life) meaſurably fortifie and ſtrengthen the Vital, Natural and Animal Spirits, it cheriſheth the principal Organs, and makes them better to perform their Office in the preparing of good Juices, for it agrees with the Callidum Innatum, *or Sulphur, as well as with the* Humidum Radicale, *or Mercury; it ſtirs up the digeſtive Faculties,*

 and

and so not only prevents from being surfeited, but also relieves from Surfeits, when Contracted; and therefore may it properly be esteemed as a rich Treasure in Families; it comforts both Young and Old; 'tis good in oppressions of Wind and Cholick, expelling the same from the Stomach and Bowels, and is also good for the Strangury and Gravel, &c.

There is not yet known or Practised by a more Excellent Medicine, both for safeness, pleasantness and speed, to expel the painful Gripes in Children, whether with or without a Looseness, which are so incident to these poor Babes, that thousands die thereof, as we may see by the weekly Bill of Mortality; therefore let such as have Children subject to Wind, or as are so themselves, make use thereof; and in few Minutes they shall find the comfortable Relief thereof; and indeed so will such as are subject to fainting and painful Diseases. 'Tis very prevalent not only to prevent Fits in Children, but also to relieve such as have them; In fine, its almost imparallel'd Virtues are such, as that we could fill pages therewith, but however shall here omit them, seeing we have been more large in the precited Book, which God willing shall ere long see the Light; seeing it may be of such publick Service in the distinguishing of the Nature of truly prepared Medicines from the common slops.

The Dose of this Cordial is from a pap Spoonful to three or four Ordinary Spoonfuls, according to the Age, Strength and Condition of the Patient; and that as often received as is requisite, which must

muſt at leaſt be three, and ſometimes five or ſix times a day, when the Patient takes little Food or Reſt.

Thus (Courteous Reader) have we with painful Labours paſſed through the Garden of Diſtillation, in which the various Flowers are to be gathered, which may be found profitable to you; the which indeed was the end of our undertaking it; that you may ſee the Nature and difference of Waters, even of the firſt, ſecond and third Order; and that you may not be deficient in any thing, which may be ſaid to appertain to this Art we ſhall ſtretch forth our Hand in our ſecond part, and ſhow you the True and Genuine way of preparing of *Vegetable Powers*, &c.

Pharmacopœa Spagyrica nova:

O R,

An *Helmontian Courſe*, wherein is laid down the true Preparation of the moſt noble and ſecret Medicines of the Ancients.

BEING

A Candid *Deſcription* of the *Triune Key*, *viz.* The Philoſophical *Sal Armoniack*, Volatile Salt of Tartar, and Spirit of our *Sal Panariſtos*, or *Great Hilech.*

TOGETHER

With their Uſe and Office in preparing *Powers*, *Arcanums*, *Magiſteries*, *Eſſences* and *Quinteſſences*, the Doſe and Virtues being annexed.

The Second Part.

By *W. Y-WORTH*, *Medicinæ Profeſſor in Doctrinis Spagyricis & per Ignem Philoſophus.*

LONDON,

Printed for J. Taylor, at the *Ship* in St. *Paul's* Church-Yard. M DCC V.

Pharmacopœa Spagyrica nova:

OR,

An Explication of Spagyrick and Specifick Medicines.

CHAP. I.

THIS *Pharmacopœa* is a choice *Archidox* of our own Experience, or an *Helmontian Course*, containing the Foundation of Specifick Medicines, prepared in a way succedaneous to the grand *Arcanums*, and only by the Knowledge of the Spagyrical Key and true *Modus* of Working, therefore did I first lay this down as a true Introduction to that.

This being founded and built on many Years Experience, through exceeding hard Labour, because with difficulty I was forced to collect them out of the Writings of the ancient Philosophers, and that understandingly; and in order to this I first began with Starkey's *Nature's Explication*, diligently tracing Helmont, and his great Master Paracelsus, Basilius, Lully, and others of the most profound Philosophers, till I came to conclude with Hermes's *Confirmation*; therefore we ſay that theſe Medicines are from thence compoſed and faithfully prepared on ſuch a Foundation as is agreeable both to Reaſon and the Law of Nature, therefore deſigned as ſecret *Noſtrums* in Practice, and not fit to be diſcovered to any but the true laborious Sons of Art.

And the principal engaging Reaſon for the Printing of theſe was, to take off that Calumny wherewith the Worthy **Helmont** is aſperſed, *viz. that he has pull'd down, but not built up*, that is, he has caſt out of Doors the common *Pharmacopœan* Medicines, but has not ſhewn the Preparation of thoſe Noble Specificks which he in his Writings ſo highly magnifies; tho' indeed the Field is ſo very large, that I may ſay they even abound, and he has written them ſo as that they may be underſtood by ſuch as will make Fire, Coles and Glaſſes their Interpreters.

But I ſhall not make long Circumlocutions in the deſcribing of many Medicines, but ſuch as are fundamental and grounded on the very Foundation of Art it ſelf, in which the ſecret *Diploma* being underſtood, they will not only ſerve as Rudiments to the Art, but alſo as the very Principles, which being known render the Profeſſor a compleat Maſter, and enable him to make Preſcriptions of his own.

Theſe here are ſo compoſed as that they will not fail to raiſe ſome Honour to this Noble Art of Healing, by letting the Sick feel the Benefit of their Virtue, for their immediate relief in acute Diſeaſes, and comforting thoſe

thoſe that are grievouſly afflicted with ſtubborn and refractory ones, diſplaying their Prevalency in rebellious Maladies; and where Life is maintain'd, tho' by never ſo faint a Power in Nature, yet will they endeavour to the utmoſt to ſtrengthen the ſame; and Life being deſigned, if they are warily adminiſtred, will always be found more ready to fortifie Nature than any other, for theſe act by an Homogeneous Affinity to that Light, and are as Fuel to her Lamp, ſtrengthening her againſt thoſe Aſſaults which are made by the darkſom diſeaſie *Ideas*, which always endeavour to dart forth their Venom and center their Points in the *Anatomia Eſſata*, or Mother of Diſeaſes, thence producing ſuch diſeaſie Off-ſprings as will endeavour to oppoſe Nature's Harmony, which Breach and Diſorder cannot be reduced into a *Tono uniſono*, or perfect Concordancy, but by that which has power to reſtore the Spirits to their priſtine and vigorous Activity, by diſſolving and caſting off the morbifick Matter, ſo as that the *Microcoſm* may come to feel and witneſs the perfect Effects of Sanity.

Such is the Nature and Virtue of many of theſe Noble Specificks, that we almoſt tremble to put them forth in this ungrateful Age, leſt their preſtant Splendor ſhould, as other Noble Medicines have been, come to be eclipſed by Sophiſtication; this being conſidered I had never ſet them forth had it not been for the gratifying of the truly Ingenious.

I ſhall therefore proceed regularly, by the way explaining and illuſtrating ſome Medicines in our **Chymicus Rationalis**, ſtating theſe things ſo as that there may e ſome Affinity between theſe and our other Labours, which (when Divine Pleaſure is) may come to Light.

Obſerve, many Medicines are here nominated, but where you ſee any notified or marked thus * you may depend that their Virtues will anſwer all that can be deſired of an Artiſt, they being the Marrow or Epitomy of the reſt; but for Ornament ſake we ſhall proceed as follows.

De Spiritibus vinariis. *Of vinous Spirits.*

The Definition of Spirits in general.

'Spirits are the ſulphureous parts of Bo-
'dies broken by Fermentation, in which Acti-
'on the volatile Atoms are united with the
'Aquoſity, and ſome Portion of the Volatile
'Salt and Mercurial Power, by Nature ripen-
'ed, and by Art ſeparated into a Spiritual
'*Ens*, containing the moſt eſſential Qualities
'of that Body whence extracted, whether
'Malted Barley, Wheat, or other Grain,
'Wine, Herbs, *&c.* according to the Defini-
'tion given in our **Firſt Part**, as alſo in
'Chap. 2. of our **Chymicus Rationalis**,
'having there handled all thoſe general Heads
'which are needful to make the Art compleat,
'and

'and therefore what I shall here add is some
'higher degrees of Improvement, and Physi-
'cal Receipts there omitted.

Now by the way observe, The principal Ground of the true Improvement and Exaltation of Spirits, is a right understanding of the Doctrine of Fermentation, that so you may obtain the full Virtue of Herbs and Flowers by proper *Mediums*, as *Molasses*, *Sugar* and *Honey*, the common Ferment being heightned by Art, which is easily done, if you understand the Preparation and Office of our **Sal Panaristos**, which will be prescribed in its proper place, for that answers all the Artist can desire in the Doctrine of Fermentation, therefore omitting to speak any further of it here shall proceed to the *Doctrine* of *Powers*, by Examples to make these things clear, and first of those of the inferior Order, *viz.*

Of Vegitable Powers:

Powers are by such a preparation only obtained as will indue them with the Strength, Force and Quality of that Concrete, whence they are prepared, that is to say, the virtuous one; for the three Principles must be united and brought to a Volatile Spirit, and here we observe, that the Abstersive Nature proceeds from the fixed Salt, the Specifick from the Sulphur and the spirituality from the Mercury; for these being in union you have the true Essentiality of the Concrete, which according to the various Preparations is is more or less exalted, for if 'tis done by the help of Urinous Spirits, it may as well be called an *Oleosum* as *Powers*, and especially if the Alkalie, contained in the Concrete, be not radically Volatized; for here is the difference between an *Oleosum* and *Powers*, as they are generally prepared, the **First** *is that, wherein Urinous Spirits are most predominant, and is made fragrant by the Vinor together with Aromatick Oyls added in the Preparations; but in the* **Latter** *the Vinor fragrancy is essentially predominant, and what Volatile or Alkalizated Spirits are therein, they are so invisible as not to be discerned*, but in the Preparation of both we observe one grand defect, which is, that although they are both spiritual, and ir Distill'd, contain many Volatile Particles of the Oyls and Spirits, insorb'd by the hidden fermentative Action of the three, yet the more solid and substantial part of the Body and Oyl is not Elevated into the Spirit, as is plainly evident in this, that there is a great quantity of Oyl and fixed Salts remaining in a ponderous Form at the bottom of the Cucurbit after the Operation is over, and the more especially if you put quantity sufficient to make *Powers* of, that is to say, a fourth, third, or half part of the *Pondus* of the whole, and yet more, if united by their fixed Salt, which cannot be truly volatilized till it hath received in three or four times its weight of Essential Oyls as will be hereafter more largely shown, but now in the defect of this you must learn to prepare Oyls, as we have men-

tion-

tioned *in our Anſwer to the* 10th. *Query of the Learned Dr.* **Boylewharſe** *in our Spagyrick Phil. Aſſerted*; that is to ſay, *they muſt be bereaved of their internal Water and floating Earth; ſo that they will readily diſſolve in and unite with Water or Spirit of Wine,* this is repeated, becauſe that Book may not come into the hands of thoſe that this doth; and further, we ſay, that Oyls may be thus very eaſily prepared by Art, ſo as to caſt forth their combuſt Earth, and as it were, an inſipid *Faces*, when as without the ſame twenty Rectifications ſhall not ſo readily perform it; and in this 'tis yet more dubious, ſeeing the Oyls by the heat of the Fire will be converted into a Combuſt Earth, remaining in the bottom of the Veſſels; and although Oyl of Vitriol, Aqua-Fort, and ſuch like Corroſives may revive part thereof, yet we look upon the Oyl to be conſiderably exhauſted, not only in *Pondus*, but alſo in Vertue; when as that which hinders their Union by a genuine Preparation is not above a tenth part; and 'tis obſervable that theſe Oyls will then unite with a fourth, third, or half *Pondus* of any truly rectified Spirit: But to perform this, is not for the *Head-wiſe Chymiſts*, but for ſuch indeed whom Experience hath made Heart-wiſe, ſeeing Nature muſt firſt graduate them with her hidden *Diploma*, which indeed is our Uniter and Reconciler of Extreams; and that we may hint how it is performed, Obſerve, Let the highly purified fixed Alkalie of any Concreate be herein diſſolved, and then pour in what quantity you pleaſe

please of its own Eſſential Oyl, digeſt and ſupply it with Oyl until the Alkalie is partly reverſed from its Saline into a Sulphurous Nature, and elevated into one Body, with the Oyl, then pour on this the fixed Salt of *Sal Anat. Lyb.* and that will immediately precipitate all the groſs parts, digeſt three, four, or five days, or until the Oyl will diſſolve in Water or Spirit of Wine, as aforeſaid, the which you may every day try; this is one good ſtep toward the Preparation of noble *Powers* and *Oleoſums*, and without it 'twill be impoſſible ever radically to unite the whole Body of the Oyl with the Spirits, whatever ſome may vainly and falſly pretend, or ever to have the Vertue of the fixed Salt elevated into the Spirit, much more one Ounce of the Body brought up into ſome Gallons of the ſame; ſo that the pretence that is in the World, of ſaying, that the Spirit is united with the fixed Salt, is a grand abuſe impoſed on the Age by *Pſeudo-Spagyriſts*: For the fixed Salt, Oyl and Spirit cannot by any way be united or reconciled, but by this *Medium*; neither can theſe be obtained in their full and Eſſential Vertues, without the benefit of its exaltative Power: Therefore let the Ingenious obſerve our words, and receive them for their Profits, as given forth; not regarding the Quacking-noiſe of thoſe who put forth ſo many Tables fill'd with the Vertue of their *Powers* and *Eſſential Spirits*, from thence drawing their Superiority to others, therein ſaying, *that they are impregnated with their fixed Salt*;

Salts; when alas! 'tis impoſſible, that the Spirit ſhould be either therewith united, or thereby exalted until truly prepared and Volatilized, as hath been ſaid; the which we are very well ſatisfied theſe Men cannot perform; for altho' their Pretences are never ſo great abroad, of doing general Service, yet when we truly conſider the thing, we know that their Ambition would be ſuch as to expoſe the *Volatile Salt of Tartar*, or any other fixed Alkalie to Sale, ſeeing the greateſt Philoſophers have laid thereon ſo great] an Applauſe, that any rational Man will believe it to be a Medicine fit and able to ſerve the Publick; but this is not to be obtained from them, neither abroad nor at home, altho' one would give ten times its weight in Gold for an Ounce thereof; we could never yet obtain one Drachm of it, altho' we have made their intimate Acquaintance our Friend in this Caſe, and therefore we ſhall but eſteem of their noiſe, as Rattles to deceive or pleaſe Fools and Children; but however, leaving this, we ſhall come to ſhow under how many Heads *Powers* and *Oleoſums* may be properly ſtated, which we ſhall only name, and ſo orderly proceed to treat thereof; under the firſt we comprehend,

Poteſtates per Hermaphroditicum Salem Ammoniacum, or Powers by the help of a prepared Sal-Armoniack: And under the ſecond, *Poteſtates nobiliſſimæ ſuccedaneæ Specificæ per ſalem Tartari Volatilem*; or, Noble Succedaneous and Specifick Powers: And under the

the third *Potestates veræ & arcanæ per salem nostrum Panaristos*, or the true essential and genuine Powers. Now these are the three Heads, under which may be comprehended all that can be said of *Powers*, we shall begin with the first, they being easiest to be prepared

Now seeing that every one cannot obtain the Volatile Salt of Tartar, neither will some indeed spend their Time or Money after it, but would rather accept of easie things; for the sake of such we shall first describe those which are made by the help of the said *Sal-Armoniack*, and how the said *Sal-Armoniack* is also to be prepared.

Those, which are made by the help of the said *Sal-Armoniack*, are of a noble and cleansing Nature, the which they borrow from the Hermaphroditical Salt, that is radically united with the Oyl and Spirit, and this in part supplies the want of the Volatile Salt of Tartar, and enriches the Powers far above those that have no Salt in them, for this Preparation, to perform it well, is no small part of the Chymical Art, and there be many of those who pretend to succedaneous Keys, that cannot do it; for the Urinous Spirit must first be bereaved of its fætor or stink, and secondly, radically united with its own purified Salt, and dried by the gentle Course of Nature, and sublimed from the Male and Female Earths, as will be shewn in the Process of *Sal-Panaristos*.

Then

Then take Oyſter-ſhels, waſh them very clean, dry them, and Calcine them to an exceeding white *Calx*, the which Powder very finely, and ſift through a fine Sieve; then take of this, and the highly purified *Sal-Armoniack*, of each a like quantity, mix them well together, and put them into a Retort, and pour thereon twice their weight of the Alkalizated Spirit of that Concrete, whence you intend to make your *Powers*, and by degrees of Fire Diſtil to drineſs, the Spirit that comes over you may rectifie from a proportionable quantity of dried Herbs, Species, or Seeds, from whence you make your *Powers* or *Oleoſum*; and then unite three pound thereof with half a pound of Eſſential Oyl by two or three Cohobations; or if your Oyl is prepared, as before directed, you may only ſhake them together and they ſhall be united; or in defect of this, you may do it by digeſtion, by adding in three or four Ounces of our *Common Reconciler*, or *Vegetable-preſerving-Salt*; and ſo have you an *Oleoſum* or *Powers* ſuperiour to any as yet by others expoſed to ſale, being not only indued with the middle Nature of the Concrete, but alſo an Abſterſive Vertue, as will be ſeen more at large hereafter; for what is here ſaid in general is ſufficient to ſignifie unto you the Preparation and Nature of thoſe *Powers* and *Oleoſums* prepared by the *Hermaphroditical Sal-Armoniack*; we ſhall therefore proceed to the Particulars, and firſt of,

Poteſtates Cinamomi, or the Powers of Cinamon.

Take of the aforeſaid prepared *Sal-Armoniack* one Pound; of the highly Alkalizated Spirit of Wine four pound, Diſtil and Unite, as before directed, then Rectifie from Cinamon, one pound moiſtned with a little Oyl of common Salt run *per del.* in a ſtrong B. M. and Cohobate two or three times upon the Cinamon, by which means its Virtue will be obtained, put this upon a pound of freſh Cinamon, and Cohobate as before, repeat this a third time, and your Spirit will become very rich of the Cinamon; now on the Cinamon that remains pour good Spirit of Wine, and extract the Tincture as long as any will come, add theſe Tinctures together, and put them into a Retort, and call off [illegible], gently dry the Extract, the Cinamon that remains after Diſtillation muſt be gently dried and Calcined into Aſhes, the which, while ſo warm as to be handled, muſt be put into a Cucurbit, pouring thereon the before mentioned Spirit, call'd over by making the Extract, put on a blind Head and digeſt three days, decant the clear, and if after that you think any Spirit remains in the Aſhes you may call it off by Diſtillation, and then with Diſtil'd Rain-water extract the Salt from the Aſhes in the Cucurbit, the which exactly filtrate, evaporate and Chriſtalize, Now add your two Spirits together.

together, and then take the Salt and extract, and grind them together with six Ounces of the Oyl of Cinamon, put them into a large Retort and pour your Spirits on them, Distil off and Cohobate three or four times, and lastly, return your Spirit back, adding in of our *Common Reconciler* four Ounces, digest four days, decant the clear, and so are the *Powers* prepared.

Their Vertues.

They are prevalent in Vertigoes, Palsies Apoplexies, Deprivation of Sense, Frensies, Madness, inveterate Pains of the Head, Megrims, sudden Coughs, Colds, and difficulty of Breathing, they not only comfort the Head and Brain, and refresh the Senses, but also cheer the Heart, resist Poison, and revive the Spirits being a powerful Medicine in Palpitations, Faintings, Swoonings, and Sickness at the Heart and Stomack, good against a stinking Breath, Indigestion and want of Appetite, and other the like Defects: They are good for vomiting and spitting of Blood, and excellent for weak and consumptive People.

They are also prevalent in the Cholick, Griping of the Guts, Wind, Pain of the Stomack and Spleen, Iliack Passion, sharp and corroding Humours in the Bowels, and all other Pains whatsoever; they cure a Diarrhea, Dysentery and Lientery, the Flux of the Liver, over-flowing of the Terms, and Whites in Women.

Their use and manner of being taken:

For Fits or any Diseases that suddenly approach; take thirty or forty drops in a Glass of Spring-water sweetned with a little Sugar, anointing the Fore-head and Temples therewith, and forcing the Savours up the Nostrils, but for Weakness and Fluxes, let forty drops be drank in a Glass of Tent two or three times a day, observe by the same Rules are made the Powers of Sassafras, and all such Woods as will yield an Essential Oyl by Distillation, all of which are more noble in vertue, than any of their common Prescriptions hitherto dispenced. The Price ten Shillings an Ounce.

Potestates Menthæ, or the Powers of Mint.

Take of Mint, gathered in the right Signature in a clear day, what quantity you please, let them be chop'd very small, or rather pounded in a great stone Mortar, and put them into a large Tun or Oyl-fat, as is ordered for Distillation, and pour thereon new Wort, or rather Mead sufficient to cover them at least an hands breadth; either of which must be blood-warm, head them well with Yeast, and let them work as we have ordered in our first part of Distillation, and after five days distil with a large Refrigeratory into *Low-wines*; the which pour again upon a fresh quantity of Mint gently dryed [the Herbs are best to be hang'd in a bag, as described

ſcribed, figure the ſecond, for ſo they will get no ill tangue] and diſtil into *proof goods*; then add freſh Herbs as before, and diſtil a third time, which is called *Rectification*; but in this we adviſe you to put in a Can or two of Water to keep the body of your Still from burning, as is uſual in *Rectification*, then rectifie from Chriſtallized Salt of Tartar, and unite it with purified *Sal-Armoniack*, and again rectifie from the Herbs in a large Cucurbit with its glaſs Helm, and ſo the Spirit becomes rich, pure, vital, ſtrong, and fragrant of the Herb; take of this three pound, of the oyl of Mint ſix ounces, and unite as directed in the generals. Obſerve that if eſſential oyls are rectified from mortified Bay-Salt, they may be brought to unite in equal *pondus* with the Spirit.

VIRTUES.

Theſe Powers are ſuperior to any of this nature hitherto extant, and wonderfully fortify the Spirits, exhilerate the Mind, ſtrengthen the Stomack, and provoke Appetite, ſtays the Hiccough and Vomiting, and ſtops the fury of cholerick Paſſions; their like prevalency is alſo ſeen in ſtopping the Flowers and Whites; externally the Temples being bathed with them eaſes the Head-ach, and cures Watry-eyes, ſtrengthening weak Sinnews, and being internally taken and externally applyed, are a Counter-poyſon againſt the venom of Serpents: The Doſe is from twenty to forty

Drops in Mead, Wine, or rather some cordial Julep made from its distil'd Water or Syrup: The Price is Twelve Pence an Ounce.

Potestates Melissæ, *or* the Powers of Bawm.

Let your Bawm be gathered in its right signature, and ordered in all things as was said of Mints, only 'tis best to add in the Fermentation a little fixed Niter, because the oleous part is not so easily manifested, as in some other Herbs, and you may make use of Sugar instead of Honey, in your fermenting, as we have directed in that of the fermentation of Flowers, Herbs, and Seeds by Sugar; but you must observe that after 'tis brought into *Proof-goods*, you must rectify at least four or five times before you Alkalizate it, or unite it with the purified *Sal-Armoniack*, and then you may proceed in all things, as in that of Mint; for the making of *Vegetable Powers*, is rather a common place than bare receipt.

VIRTUES.

[illegible] are a great Comforter of the Heart, [illegible] cold and moist Stomacks, and thence help Concoction, they imbibe evil Fumes, and so [illegible] open the Brain, but also strengthen and [illegible] they cure the Tooth-ach, penetra-[illegible] Blood in the Kings's-evil, Scurvy, [illegible], Jaundice and Worms, they

expel

expel Poyson and the Plague, and cure the biting of Mad-dogs; they so wonderfully fortify the vital and natural Spirits, that a certain Author says, they are endued with renovating virtue, even to restore old Age to a youthful strength, but whether so or not, we can't say, but this we know, by Experience, that they revive the most melancholy Person into a wonderful cheerfulness, and are also excellent, being externally used, for hard Swellings and the Gout, and to bath grieved parts: The Dose is from fifteen to thirty drops, sometimes forty, according to age and strength, in a Glass of Ale, Mead, or any fragrant Wine, you may give them thrice a day; the price is fourteen pence an ounce.

Potestates Sambuci Succinatæ, or the Powerful united Spirit of Elder Essentificated with Amber.

Take the Berries when ripe, and pick out the stalks and green ones, and with a large Press, as for Apples, press out their Juice, cask it up with a little Bay-salt and sweets or stumme, and in a warm place cause them well to ferment; you may let them have some Age; and then refine down with Izing-glass and rack off, so you will have a Noble Wine, as you were show'd in the first part; then on the Cheese or Berries that remain you may pour Rain or Spring-Water, and press a second time, and boil the Liquor half an Hour, and then putting it into the Receivers let it ſtand till about Blood warm, and to every Gallon add a Pound of Sugar, ſtir them well together, and with Ale Yeſt ſet it as you do a Back, and after five days diſtil with a Refrigeratory into *Low-Wines*, *Proof-Goods*, and *Rectified Spirits*, by the third Extraction, then take freſh Berries and fill an Earthen Pan therewith, and after the Bread is drawn ſet them in the Oven, and then preſs forth their Juice, to every Pound of which add a Pound of Six-penny Sugar, and boiling it into a Syrup clarifie it with Whites of Eggs, then to every Gallon of the ſaid Wines add a Pound of the ſaid Spirit, and two Pounds of the Syrup or Sweets, and let them ferment, but obſerve to row them well together as you put them in, and ſo will you have a *Noble Wine Royal of Sambucus*, endued with noble Virtues, as we have ſaid in our firſt Part; now this muſt be again diſtill'd into *Low-Wines* and *Proof-Spirits*, and then rectified from the Flowers ſeaſonably gathered until it is a Sulphur wholly inflamable; it will be yet the purer if you rectify it from its own Salt drawn from the Aſhes of the Wood burnt; now that Salt volatilized, and an Oil drawn from the dry Wood, and theſe three united was formerly our *Powers*, but to ſuccinate it proceed thus: Take of the beſt Amber three Pound, and diſtil in a glaſs Retort by the degrees of Fire, ſeparate the Spirit from the Oil, and rectify the Oil from Spirit of Salt, or *A. R.* as we have ſhown in the Chapter of Oyls in our *Chym. Rational.* And then from the dryed

Wood

Wood of Elder macerated with Bay-ſalt in a large Refrigeratory, and ſo you have a noble tranſparent Oyl, the which reſerve 'till hereafter; now the Spirit and Salt of Amber you muſt mix with equal parts of purified *Sal-Armoniack*, and by means of the aforeſaid Oyſter-ſhels force them into a Spirit, which being rectifyed is in it ſelf *a moſt noble Medicine*, and being united with common Tartarized Spirit of Wine, *will perform more than that which is made from Flowers of Sal-Armoniack ſublimed from common Salt, both in its Philoſophical uſe in drawing Tinctures, as alſo its Medicinal Virtues*: Now take of the aforeſaid Spirit of Elder ſeven pound, of the ſuccinated Spirit of purified *Armoniack*, even now taught one pound, and of the aforeſaid Oyl of Amber twelve ounces, and of our *Common Reconciler* ſix ounces, ſhake them well together and they ſhall be united, and digeſting four days, decant the clear, and thus are the *Noble Succinated Powers of Elder* Prepared.

Obſerve, I thought it convenient to give this at large for two Reaſons, the firſt is, that if the ſhell of the Berry is fermented, inſtead of relieving the Animal Faculties, it will toxicate the Brain like Man-drake or Hen bane; the ſecond is, the Oyl being hard to prepare without our *Sal Panariſtos*, therefore have we added the Oyl of Amber, which Magnetically attracts it out of the wood; we have ſeen the Effect of the former by ſuch who have made the Spirits by fermentation, without expreſſing the Juice; therefore have we given this caution.

VIR-

VIRTUES.

This is a most excellent and praise-worthy Medicine, far beyond that set forth in our **Britanean Magazine of Liquors,** *both for internal and external uses, 'tis prevalent for most Diseases incident to the Body, especially for Agues and Feavers, Surfeits, Pains in the Head or Back, Vomiting, Gripes and Looseness; 'tis a safe and powerful Medicine in the Jaundice, Scurvy, and Dropsie, Gout and Stone, and several other Diseases, as will be seen by its Use and Dose.*

In all Acute Diseases you may take from forty to fifty drops every three hours in a glass of Sack mull'd with Cinamon, and swating plentifully in Bed thereon, wonderful Relief will be found, for the offending Matter will be carried off by Sweat and Urine.

In Pestilential Diseases, such wherein the Mass of Blood is corrupted, as Small-pox, Swine-pox, Measlles, &c. You must take it five or six times a day in a Glass of Sack Posset-drink, wherein Saffron is braid, and so the Venom will be carried from the Heart, and the Vital Spirits be strengthned, and as the Disease begins to abate, purge two or three times with the Golden Spirit, to carry off the Reliques of the same.

For Gripes and tormenting pains of the Wind, Cholick, Strangury, and want of Rest, make a Brandy Caudle, and as it is fit to drink put in at least sixty drops, sweat well in Bed and admirable Relief will be found.

&c.

For the Phthisick, shortness of Breath, Consumption, Dropsie, Scurvy, and Stone in the Bladder, you must take forty drops every six hours in the Juice of baked Turnips clarified, and as much of its own Syrup as will serve to make it into a Cordial, whose use must be continued until Relief is found; this also does excellent well in the Gout, and for Ricketty, Consumptive Children; as also for Sprains, Bruises and Squatts, only let the spirit without any mixtion be externally used, and chafe the grieved part therewith.

In fine, its Virtues are so excellent, that we advise all Sea-faring-men never to be without some Bottles of it, for 'twill not only preserve them from such Diseases as are incident to them, as Scurvy, Calenture, Loathings, Gripes, &c. *but also ease and cure them of the same, being taken in Water sweetned with its own Syrrup, or a little Sugar, in which Cases the ordinary Dose is from thirty to sixty drops, according as the Strength and Age of the Patient is :* The Price of our first *Powers* of *Elder*, is one Shilling the Ounce-bottle, but of these, one Shilling and Six Pence.

Observe, Mine is only to be had at my House, because there is a nameless Bill put forth by one *Andrew Sole*, who hath made use of most of my words out of my Receipt given in our *Britanean Magazine*, and therefore I thought it convenient to signific that I cannot own his Spirit, much less his proceedings, seeing 'tis great imprudence in him to ascribe to himself that which his Experience can't demonstrate the hundreth part of.

Pote-

Poteſtates Roſmarini, or the Powers of Roſemary.

Take the Leaves of Roſemary gathered in the right ſignature and dryed, and put them into a large *Matrix*, and caſt thereon four or five handfuls of fine *Calx vive*, and gently ſtir them together, if your quantity is large it muſt be more, even a third part of the weight of the Herb, then pour thereon Rain-water diſtil'd from its *Faeces*, after forty days putrifaction, and diſtil off about two thirds, and you will have a *Low-wine* very pregnant and ſtrong of the Herb, then take the like quantity of Roſemary and put it into the diſtil'd Rain-water, juſt enough for the Water to cover, and putting on a blind head decoct it thirty hours in *Balneo*, let this be put blood-warm upon an other quantity of Roſemary leaves, Flowers and all, and the aforeſaid *Low-wines* already diſtil'd off, and adding a pound of Sugar to every gallon, ſtir them well together, head them well with Yeſt, and let them ferment five days, diſtil again a ſecond time into Proof-goods, and adding freſh Roſemary with a little Bay-ſalt, bring it into rectified Spirits, and a fourth time make it fine by rectifying from freſh Herbs and equal parts of the Oyl of its own fixed Salt run *per del.* Tartar, or any other fixed Alkaly, then unite two pound of this with one pound of the highly purified *Sal-Armoniack* by the help

help of the aforesaid *Calx*, and add this to a gallon of the aforesaid prepared Spirit, put it into a great Cucurbit, and fill as full as you can with Flowers, and let it stand close luted in the Sun for five days, then put on the Alembick with its Receiver and distil, and you will have a volatile, subtil, and fragrant Spirit, which quantity being united with a pound of the Oyl, as was directed in the other *Powers*, you have the true *Powers* of *Rosemary*.

Their Virtues.

This is indeed a Medicine of praise-worthy Vertues, far superiour to the slop Hungarian Water *sold, being prevalent against most Diseases of the Head, Stomack, Heart, Womb, or any other Viscera, it may be applyed to any Disease of the Head, especially Apoplexy, Epilepsy, Convulsions and Vertigoes, the weakness of Nerves, Head-ach, hardness of Hearing, and dimness of Sight, it comforts the Head and Brain, refreshing the Animal Spirits, and clearing the Vital ones, therefore good against all Palpitations, Faintings, Swoonings, and Fits of the Heart, neither doth it forget to do its part toward the natural Spirits, for it opens the Obstructions of the Liver, Spleen, Womb, and so cures Agues, Feavers, Scurveys, Jaundice, and several other Diseases as will be seen by its Use and Dose.*

For any of the aforesaid Diseases, you must take from twenty or thirty drops, three or four times a day in a Glass of Mead or Wine, that is, an hour before

before each meal; but for the Gripes of the Guts, Cholick, Oppression of Wind, or sharp Acrimonious Humours in the Spirits or Bowels, you must take sixty drops in a Glass of mull'd Sack in the Paroxisms, repeating it every three hours till relief is found: For Agues you must take the largest dose an hour before the fit, and soundly sweat thereon; 'tis also good to be given thus in mull'd Wine both before and after Delivery to facilitate the Birth, and to ease After pains: It is observeable to us that it is an Health-preserving Medicine, keeping People lively that take it: But for old Aches, the Gout, Rheumatism, Pains and Weakness of Sinews and Nerves, the Palsy and Cramp, violent Head achs, and dimness of sight, you must externally strike the grieved parts therewith two or three times a day, taking the Savours up the Nostrils; if you wash the Face therewith 'tis an excellent Cosmetick, clearing and beautifying the Skin, The Price is Twelve Pence an Ounce.

Observe, thus may be prepared the Powers *of* Pennyroyal and others.

Potestates Cochleariæ, or the Powers of Scurvey grass.

Take Scurvey-grass-wine, the Preparation of which is shown in our *Britanean Magazine* of Liquors, or else in place of that, take Scurvey-grass in *May*, *June* or *July*, when it is in its Flowers, and stamp it in a stone Mortar, and put it into a large Tun, and pour thereon as much Liquor blood-warm, in which *Molasses*

Molasses or Honey is dissolved, as will just cover them, head them well with Yeast, and set them to ferment, and after four days distil into *Low-wines*, and *Proof-Spirits*: Observe that the Fermentation is promoted by an Onion dipt in strong Mustard, and a Ball of Whiting cast in, this will bring a Tun of Molasses-goods forward when defective in working; *Argell* does well to give an internal Ferment, it also moderates and flats a Tun when too violent; now being brought into *Proof-goods*, you must take Scurvy-grass, which hath been compressed with Christals of Tartar or Salt, Hony or Molasses in a close Tub smeered over with Barm, but no Liquor must be put to it; and having stood three days in a cold place, for in a warm one we have observed that much of the *Crasis* will be lost, which consists in a Volatile Armoniack, put it into your Still as full as you can cram, and then pour thereon the aforesaid Aireal Spirit, for 'tis far superiour to Spirit of Wine, which too too much many use, enough to cover or moisten them just to the top, close the Head of your Still very exactly, and let your Recipient be so, as that no Air may come in; give it for the first day a ferment in the Still, and the second Distil, but as it begins to work, you must damp your Fire very close, for it must come but softly, so let it run as long as any goodness comes; you must repeat this Operation a second and third time with fresh Grass, and if you add in a little *Volatile Salt of Tartar, or Sal Anotasier Lybianus*, and have

a

a Pewter head you may Diſtil, and receive a part as long as it runs all Fire; the after running you may ſave for a freſh beginning: Obſerve, when you think that you have too much Flegm in the Still you may add a quantity of *decrepitated Bay-ſalt*, and ſo will it be deflegm'd. The way to make the Spirit purging is ſhown in our *Chymicus Rationalis*; but for the *Powers* proceed thus; take Scurvy-graſs and ſmeer it over with new Muſtard, and lay a lay of that, and another of Scurvy-graſs-ſeed, ſo continue *ſtr. ſup. ſtr.* and ſmeer up the uppermoſt alſo with Muſtard, ferment with Water and Salt, and diſtil into Eſſential Oyl, the way is ſhown in our *Chymicus Rat.* then being ſeparated unite one pound of this with ſix pound of the Spirit, according to the way directed in other *Powers*; and ſo are they prepared.

Their Virtues.

Theſe Powers are abundantly ſurpaſſing in Virtue any other Preparation of Scurvy-graſs whatſoever, and as I formerly told you, they were originally prepared by me in Holland, *and preſented to both Univerſities, which for goodneſs, ſtrength, and pleaſantneſs of Taſt were allowed to ſtand parallel with, nay, ſome were of opinion that they clearly out-ſtripped thoſe of the greateſt* Pretenders *in* Europe, *the* **Modus Operandi**, *of which I never ſo plainly before communicated; but I have now done it on purpoſe to be ſerviceable to the ingenious, and to deſtroy the uſe of that ſophiſticated*

sticated Spirit sold, which is made in six or eight hours time, with a little Malt Spirit and Scurvy-grass, made burning and sharp in tast with Horse-radish, but this Spirit is not to be valued; for 'tis impossible to take out the Specifick Virtue of the Grass without an higher Exaltation, and the reason why the sick are often disappointed in their Expectation is this, the slight Preparation that many Pretenders make, for the Grass will not so easily give forth its central Virtue, for this, when truly obtained, hath an excellent effect in relieving from many Diseases, and principally the Scurvy, because the Herb hath a signature against the Disease, it helps the Liver, Spleen, and other Viscera in their Defects; it fortifies the vital Spirits, and gives Circulation to the Blood, its internal texture being made up of a Volatile Armoniack, and Vinor Essence united with a vital medicinal Crasis, and as the Learned Physicians allow, as well Modern as Ancient, which that worthy Mrs. Experience *daily confirms, there is no Herb in the Vegetable Kingdom of a more Specifick Virtue in curing the Scurvy, than the aforesaid Scurvy-grass, for 'tis a great Abstersive, and so dissolves and dissipates congealed Humours, for by its Alkalisated Nature it opens and mundifies, and by its Vinor are the Venoms embibed and destroyed, so by its carrying off all the Saline crude Humours which are the original Cause of the Scurvy, whether proceeding from living in crude moist and foggy Airs, where the Sea-damps are, or from raw sowr Fruits, or exceeding Salt Fish or Flesh, as is plainly demonstrated by the incident of the Disease upon*

Seafaring-persons, especially such as use long Voyages, it sweetens the Blood; this Spirit doth not only cure this Disease in all its Symptoms, but also prevents it from approaching in such as take it for prevention sake, therefore in brief, what we have to say is, that it is indued with virtue to give Sanity to the principal Faculties. and is a certain Specifick both at Sea and Land where this popular Disease Reigns; as also in Camps and Armies against the Chilbane and Rot, which are usually there, by which Men dye as Chore-sheep.

Their Use and Dose.

For the Scurvey, Jaundice, Dropsie, Consumtion, Phthisick, or shortness of Breath, these Powers may be used at all times, the oftner the better, the Dose is ten, twenty, thirty or forty drops according to the Age, Strength, and Constitution of the Patient, in a Glass of Wine, Beer, Tea, or Coffee, as best liked, The Price is one Shilling an Ounce.

Now according to these Rules you may take any *Vegetable Powers*, therefore we shall omit instancing such as depend on common places, and come to give a description of such as are Compound.

Potestates Emundantes, or our General Cleansing Powers.

Take of Venice-Turpentine four pound, Tartarized Spirit of Wine the like quantity, and

and put them into a large Retort, diſtil, and there will aſcend a Spirit and fragrant Oyl, as we have ſhown in making the Eſſential Oyl of Turpentine in our *Chymicus Rationalis*; the Oyl muſt be made Aireal by rectifying ſeveral times from Bay-ſalt, as is alſo there ſhown; the Spirit you muſt pour on Frankincenſe, and Maſtick of each two ounces, Aloes Hepatick, Date-ſtones, Laudanum, Caſtor, the Roots of Bettony, and Elecampane, of each an ounce and an half, Cardamums, Cloves, Nutmegs, Ginger, Galingal, Cubebs, Calamus Aromaticus, Lignum Aloes, Yellow-Saunders, Zedoary, Pepper, Spiknard, Lawrel-berries, Smallage-ſeeds, Mug-wort-ſeeds, Sweet-fennel-ſeeds, Ani-ſeed, Sorrel-ſeeds, of each two ounces and an half, the Flowers of Braſil, red and white Roſes of each three ounces, Germander, Tormentil, Juniper-berries, Agrimony, Centaury, Fumitory, Pimpernel, Dandelion, Eye-bright, Feverfew, of each two ounces, Rhubarb three ounces, dried Figs, Raiſins, Sweet Almonds, of each four ounces, Virgins Hony ſix pound, *Mevis* Sugar ten pound; to theſe add of our Fermentative Salt three ounces, and being cloſe luted digeſt in the heat of Horſe-dung twenty days in the Veſſel deſcribed, fig. 4. Then take out, and clapping on an head with its Receiver, lute all faſt and diſtil in *B* 'till all is over that will aſcend, which firſt will come in a white Spirit, ſecondly more deep, and thirdly a yellowiſh red with ſome floating Oyl, which fragrant

Spirit and Oyl preſerve and unite with the aforeſaid Etherial Oyl of Turpentine ; ob-ſerve, you may remove your Veſſel out of the *B.* into a Sand or Reverberatory Furnace, and by degrees of Fire force over all that will come, which will be a ſtinking Flegm with ſome fetid Oyl, the which may be rectifyed from Spirit of Salt, as we have taught in our *Chymicus Rationalis*, and ſo it will become fragrant and fit to be united with the Medi-cine; then take of Musk, and Amber-greece three ounces, and Cohabate in *B.* two or three times till united, and laſtly, force all over till dry in the bottom ; the ſubtil Spirit carefully preſerve out of the *fæces* that remains in the bottom, you muſt extract the Tincture with highly Rectified Spirit of Cinamon, as long as it tinges the Spirit, all which ſaid Tinctures put together and Filtrate ; and putting it in *Baln.* adapt a Receiver, lute cloſe and call off two thirds, the which may be put away for other uſes ; then evaporate the Flegm unto the conſiſtence of an Extract, the which add to your Medicine, and digeſt with three oun-ces of fine Sugar till united, and if any thing precipitate, decant the clear, the which care-fully preſerve for uſe.

VIRTUES.

Theſe Powers are a noble Medicine, carrying a ſuperiority of Virtue with them, anſwering all that is attributed to the Powers of Turpentine, the Stone-powers, and others ; but if you eſteem of of Cantharides, Hog-lice, and dried Toades distiled by violence of Fire, and then rectified and united, you may take them for me, and I'll administer these, altho' we confess that if these were dissolved by the volatile and genuine Spirit of Tartar, or having respect to Glauber *in his prescription for the Stone, which is prepared by his wonderful* Sal Mirabilis, *much might be expected therefrom; for we know that a Toad, altho' so great a poyson, may by these be so prepared, as to deserve the name of an* Arcanum *in the Plague, far above any hitherto known in the World; but this being treated of in its proper place, shall be omitted here, and so proceed to speak of the excellent virtue of these Powers, which indeed are profitable in many Diseases, especially in the Strangury, or difficulty of making Water, Stone, Gravel, Sand, or Slime, and such offensive things which obstruct the Urinary passage; they open Obstructions and highly provoke Urine, being very profitable in all kind of Fluxes, excellent in Fevers, Agues, Jaundice, Scurvy, Leprosy, and all foulness and corruption of Blood; externally used, they cure new and green Wounds, tho' in the Nerves, old Aches, Ulcers, tho' never so rebellious; they are excellent for* Noli-me-tangere's, *and Plague-sores, Impostumes and Fistula's, they ease the Gout, and are helpful in Rheumatisms, Palsie, and weakness of Members; they are good in the Hemmorrhoids or Piles, and many other Diseases, for they will perform all that can be expected of a Medicine short of succedanous ones.*

Their way of being taken.

You may take from fifteen to twenty drops, mornings only in a glass of Rhenish wine sweetned with the Syrup of Marsh-mallows, but strong Constitutions may take thirty or forty: For external uses, where any grief is, you must bath the part till relief is found; for Sore-eyes, or those that have a Pearl, you must drop in a drop once in two days; but for Wounds and Ulcers, you must dip a pledge therein and apply it with some proper Plaister.

The Price is 2 *s.* 6 *d.* an Ounce.

Potestates Nepenthe, or our Annodyne Pain-easing Powers.

Take Poppies gathered in their right signature, and in a cold Still, Distil the Water therefrom, then take fresh Poppy leaves, and putting them into a Matrix strow them over with the *Calx vive*, after the same manner as directed in making *Potestates Rosmarini*, distil off about ⅔ thereof, ferment with Sugar, distil into Low-wine, and from fresh Flowers rectify into *Proof-goods*, and by reiteration into *fine Spirits*; then take a large quantity of Poppy-seeds, which by Art must be macerated, and so distil into Essential Oyl, then take of the best *Theban* Opium, and with the aforesaid Spirit extract all the Tincture, and make an Extract, as before directed, and to every three

three pound of the Spirit you call over, add one pound of the aforesaid purified *Sal-Armoniack*, and a pound of the prepared *Calx* of Oyster-shells, and macerate them together with the *Faeces* of the Opium that was left of the Extract, put them into a Retort, and by violence of Fire force over all that will come, the which preserve, and the *Faeces* that are in the Retort, set in a cold moist Cellar to run *per deliquium*, the which exactly filtrate and Christallize, and you will have a noble Opiated Salt, take the whole quantity of this Salt, and of Cinamon ten ounces, Nutmegs, Cloves, and broad Mace of each four ounces, macerate them and put them into a Retort, and pour the aforesaid Spirit on them, and distil in *B.* to dryness, then take this Spirit so prepared and aromatized, and equal parts of the first Spirit, put them together, and add in the Extract, and Camphire one ounce, of the Narcotick Sulphur of *Venus* six ounces, and of the aforesaid Essential Oyl eight ounces, digest till united, which will easily be if you proceed by Cohobation, and Digestion, as before directed.

These are wonder-working Powers, and perform more than we are willing to put upon them; being far above any Liquid Laudanum hitherto extant to the World, and more prevalent in any Disease to which that is attributed; for by this method is the Opium well corrected and brought to a safe and pleasant Medicine, prevalent against Spitting of Blood, Catarrhs, Fluxes of any kind, Terms, Whites, and Gonorrhea's, as also in Restlesness,

Watchings, and Fevers, Melancholy, Frensy, Epilepsy, Convulsion, and Fits of the Mother, Plurisy, Vomiting, and Cholick, there is hardly a better Remedy to be found for any violent Pain or Restlesness in the Body, whatever vain Applauses too too many fill Books with, who make as if one Medicine should be Universal against all Diseases; but our Knowledge of Nature hath learned us so much the contrary, that we have a perfect abhorrence against this canting way, however our limitations being given in other Writings, we shall omit it here: The Dose is from three to five, from thence to twenty drops in some Cordial Julep, according to the strength of the Disease, and Age and Constitution of the Patient. The Price is 2 *s.* 6 *d.* an Ounce.

Potestates Baccarum Juniperi, or the Powers of Juniper-berries.

Take of Juniper-berries twenty or thirty pound, or what quantity you please, pound them small, and putting them into a Tub pour thereon Rain-water, adding thereunto an handful of Bay-salt, and so let them stand ten or twelve days, and then distil in a Copper-still with a Refrigeratory, so that pure Oyl will ascend with Water in good quantity; and when the Liquor and Berries are taken out of the Still, if you press through an hair-bag, filtrate and evaporate, you shall find good quantity of Extract, and yet the more, if they have had a Ferment by some Gummous and Vinous-Nature,

ture; the Water that comes over must be separated from the Oyl by a separating Glass, and then distil'd over again with fresh Berries and *Calx vive*, as directed in other *Powers*, and so brought to *Low-wines*, *Proof-goods*, and *Rectified Spirits*, by adding in fresh Berries to enrich the same; now some talk of drawing the Calcin'd Salt out of the Berries, but we, as an Operator, tell you that the quantity will be so insignificant, as not to be worth your Fire and Time spent about it, as upon Tryal you will find; if it is to cleanse your Spirit, Salt of Wormwood, or Tartar will do the same: But to talk of Volatizing this, or any other fixed Alkaly in a whiff, is stuff; for 'tis not to be performed under Ten Weeks or Three Months, and that by the hand of a Skilful Philosopher, and then only by essential Oyls, and so it takes on it the tast and smell of that Oyl by which it is Volatized, and hath all the Power Strength, and Force of the Concrete, so that it is no matter what the Alkaly is, and therefore have not *Starkey* and *Helmont* in vain called *Tartar the publick Family of Alkalies*; but we will not teach you here such difficulties, but advise you to the Hermaphroditical Salt before described, one pound whereof is to be united with two of the Spirit by Distillation, then that with a gallon of the other Spirits, and a pound of the Essential Oyl, as was directed in other Powers, so are they prepared, being tinged by their own Extract.

These

These Powers are of great Service in the Cholick, Gripes, Oppressions of Wind, and Gravel in the Kidneys, Ureters, and Bladder, they not only ease violent pains, but also open the Obstruction of parts, they prevalently provoke Urine, comfort the Stomack, Bowels and all the Viscera, the vital Spirits receive the Benefit thereof, it is a general Custom in Holland, *when the Child is troubled with Oppressions of Wind, for the Mother whilst the Child is sucking, to drink of the Powers or Spirit of Juniper, by which the Child is Relieved; what shall I say more than this, we know that the Powers are indued with the virtue of the Juniper-berry let it be by what manner soever prepared, so that we leave the rest to the discretion of the Ingenious: The Dose is as of other Powers, from fifteen to forty drops, in a Glass of Beer, Wine or Mead, for complicate Diseases they may be variously mixed with other Powers, and principally for violent Pains, with our Potestates Nepenthe.* The Price 1 *s.* an Ounce

Now by these Rules may be made the *Powers* of any Berries whatsoever, nay, from what is here said and laid down, you may comprehend whatever belongs to *Vegetable Powers*: And as to *Urinous Powers*, their Preparation, Use, and Dose, is described in our *Chymicus Rationalis*, and *Spagyrick Philosophy Asserted*, under the Title of *Oleosums* and *Powers*, so that it would be but fruitless Repetitions to insert them here.

Po-

Poteſtates Coſmeticæ, or our Beautifying Powers.

Take of Bean-flowers five handfuls, *Nants* Brandy two quarts, digeſt them fourteen days in the Sun, and Diſtil; then add thereunto of the Roots of white Lillies gently dried, Aron-roots, Fenugreek, Contra yerva, *Virginia* Snake-root, of each four ounces, Spurge three ounces, Pimpernel, Roſemary, and Celendine of each two ounces, Camphire one ounce, and diſtil *S. A.* Then take of this one pound, of the Oyl of Talk deſcribed in our *Chym. Rat.* two ounces, digeſt them till united, and ſo are the *Powers* prepared.

Their Virtues and Uſe.

Theſe being Externally uſed, are powerful in taking off all enormities of the Skin, wonderfully beautifying the ſame, and by the right uſe thereof Freckles, Sunburn, Pimples, and Scurf will vaniſh, they make the Skin ſo truly Smooth, and Beautiful, that Wrinkles and Old Age are hardly diſcernable; But obſerve that you clean the Face well before you uſe it, you may either rub your Face with it alone, or mixed with White-wine, which you pleaſe The Price is from one to five Shillings an Ounce, according as it is exalted with the Oyl of Talk.

Po-

Poteſtates Mercurii, or our Powers of Mercury.

The Preparation hereof we have faithfully diſcovered in our *Chym. Rat.* under the Title of the *Oyl* of *Mercury*, together with their Virtue; *being moſt prevalent in the Scurvy, Gout. Pox, Leproſie and Itch; but we think it convenient to add, that they are alſo an excellent Coſmetick, taking off Tetters, Herpes, Scabs and Pocky Eruptions, and for perſons that are very Tawny, they are neceſſary to be uſed before our* **Poteſtates Coſmeticæ**: *Spring-water proceeding from a good Chalk-well, is as good a Vehicle or Dilative as can be, therefore we need not preſcribe another.* The Price is 7 *s.* 6 *d.* an Ounce.

Now having given the gradual Preparation of ſeveral noble Medicines, in our *Chym. Rat.* and largely explained the Specifick in our *Spagyrick Phyloſophy's Triumph,* we ſhall thither refer you for your Satisfaction, and we are almoſt perſwaded, that you will not think your Money, Labour and Time in reading them loſt: But that you, if you put your hand to the Plow, and come experimentally to know and witneſs the Miſteries therein contained, will then only value them according to their deſerved Merit, ſo leaving the whole to your judicious Conſideration, hoping that this at preſent will ſuffice concerning

ing *Powers* of this order, we ſhall proceed to touch at thoſe in general, which are of a more ſuperiour one.

CHAP. II.

The Authors Letters to J. M. Practitioner *of* Surgery *and* Phyſick, *ſhewing the true Diſtinction between true* Oleoſums, *and thoſe ſo called; and therefore added for the Benefit of the true Deſirer, and for the undeceiving of the deceived, as an Introduction to the* Doctrine *of* Oleoſums *and* Powers, *being both pertinent and ſuitable to that Subject.*

SIR,

I Had not in the leaſt concerned my ſelf with your Medicine, had you not given it the Name of *the Genuine Medicine of the Antient Philoſophers*; and to confirm the ſame for a Truth to the World, you ſay, *'tis too evident to be confuted by the Artifice of any.* But then conſequently it muſt bear the Eſſays which the Antients have aſſign'd theirs, and which we find Recorded in the Writings of **Paracelſus, Helmont** and **Starkey**; if not an eaſie Artifice will confute it, *viz.* The bring-

in

ing it to the Probe, and if it ſtands not the Teſt it confutes it ſelf, and ſhews that the Author has falſly put an extravagant *Encomium* on it, a common Fault which the *Oleoſum*-mongers are frequently guilty of.

One ſays, that his is the *Oleoſum* of the Antients, another, that his is ſuch a Secret, ſtnatch'd out of the Boſom of Nature, and that by a kind of Providence, as but one in an Age is found worthy of: And thus by your Arrogancy, Aſſuming true Names to falſe Medicines, you ſeek to out-vie each other.

Now whether the Curing of Diſeaſes is the true Proof, which you ſeem to make the Proof of yours, where you ſay *It ſo apparently and undeniably diſtinguiſhes it ſelf from all others*, that *Numbers can* add *Teſtimonies of its* noble *Effects* in *thoſe* very *Caſes*, which *before* had *baffled*, *even* that (*among others*) of the *Diſpitous* [or Spiteful] *Pretender*, further aſſerting, *that* as a *Medicine in all Cronick Diſeaſes*, it *ſo* clearly *vindicates it ſelf* in *diſplaying its Virtues*, that *thoſe who once take* it *will never be miſlead* by *the* Name, *ſince they can be ſupplyed with the thing*, &c. I ſay, whether this be the true Proof, I ſhall conſider, and Diſſecting your Advertiſement, ſhall anſwer every Particular, as it will bear without the leaſt Strain or Force.

In the firſt place, as to the Name, if your Medicine is not true, 'tis a groſs and ignorant Impoſition on the World, and the higheſt Abuſe that can be offer'd to the Antients, or or their Writings little leſs than Sacriledge to rob the Dead of their Honour, putting a Slop in lieu of a true Medicine: Indeed by what follows, you think you make ſure, that your Medicine is too evident in its diſtinguiſhing Virtues, to be refuted; but your Proof for this, *viz.* That Numbers can teſtifie of its Effects, ſeems to me very weak; for 'tis too evident, that the ignorant are too much impoſed on, not only by the Names of Medicines, but alſo in the Nature of Diſeaſes; for they themſelves can judge equally as well of the Nature of a Diſeaſe, as a blind Man can of Colours, and 'tis too much the ſubtil Artifice of the fallaceous Pretenders to make acute Chronick, and Chronick Refractory and Stubborn; nay, ſometimes Symptoms they make Branches, and the Branches themſelves Roots; and this only to magnifie the Vertue of their Medicines, when all the while they may be as ignorant as the deluded Patient: What the true Nature of the Diſeaſe is, whether Acute, Chronick, Refractory or Hereditary; which laſt, as it comes Originally in the Seed, becomes habitual; ſo that many of them are not in the leaſt Mortal (tho' often very painful and troubleſome) and thoſe that do kill, kill only by length of time; and many of them are ſo Refractory, as not to be reach'd by any Specifick or Arcanum, ſhort of the grand Medicine, or *Panacea* of the Antients,

So that it may be reaſonably concluded, that neither the Patients, nor ſingle Practitioner's oner's Evidence is ſufficient, to prove or lay down the Nature and Difference of Diſeaſes under their true Head; the Learned themſelves being ſo often miſtaken in this Point; therefore no Authority can prove a Diſeaſe ſuch, but that of a *Quorum* of Phyſitians, who are Learned and Approved in the Knowledge of Diſeaſes; ſo that what you aſſert on this Head, is no Demonſtration at all; and we commonly ſee, that many ſimple and innocent old Womens Medicines, when rightly adapted, do cure many Refractory Diſeaſes.

Another Conſideration is upon the word [All] Chronick Diſeaſes, which at once ſhews the very Mark of an Impoſtour, for all true Phyſitians allow, that every Diſeaſe paſſing the Revolution of the Moons Monthly Motion, or twenty eight Days, making then a new Motion, becomes Chronick, and looſes the Name of Acute; ſo that all Diſeaſes being comprehended under the Names of Acute and Chronick, the Refractory and Hereditary muſt of conſequence come under the latter, ſome of which, as I ſaid before are Incurable, and not to be reach'd by any thing, ſhort of the *Elixir Vitæ*: So that the word [All] plainly ſhews the Author's Ignorance, in the Nature of many ſtubborn Diſeaſes, as alſo in the Art of Medicine, for every true and Succedaneous Medicine bears the Name of Specifick, and they are (as being appropriated by the God of Nature) for the Cure of ſuch and ſuch Diſeaſes only, which they

will

will effect, when even Refractory, and yet will not in the least touch the Root of a contrary Disease. So that Medicines of this Rank borrow the Name, *Specifick*, from their Nature and Vertue, being only appropriable to some certain and particular Diseases.

Of this Number is *the Genuine Oleosum of the Antients*, or *Volatile Salt of Tartar*, for that it is only, which deservedly bears the Name, and is the very thing without deceit of Names, carrying with it for its true Proof a Mechanick Demonstration, as well as Medicinal Vertue: The Mechanical is not only manifest in its Preparation, but also in its Office and Effect, when prepared. In its Preparation it is the *fixed Salt* of *Tartar*, truly Volatized by *Essential Oyls*, and *Vinous* and *Urinous Spirits*; in such a way, as that the Salt shall drink in at least three or four, nay, if the Artist pleases, six times its weight of Oyl, and thirty two times its weight of Spirit of Wine, in and through which Actions all shall be Salified, giving forth only a small quantity of Resinous Gum, insipid Flegm, and a foul Earth; the whole then being Distillable in a Fire of the third Degree, as *Spirit* of *Nitre*, or *Spirit* of *Salt*; and in this you have the true Vertue of the whole Body of Salt and Oyl, fragrant, yet very different from those Volatile and slight *Oleosums*, now a days made; for these have only the Light and Volatile Parts of the Saline, Oleous and Urinous Spirits ascend, the Essential and seminal Parts remaining below, fixed and united, in which only consists the Specifick Vertue for the Cure of Chronick and Refractory Diseases for bodily Spirits only have Power to reach fixed Diseases, yet not all, but such only as they are appropriated to.

Another Principal, Mechanical and Mathematical Demonstration, the sole, true and only Proof of *the Oleosum* of *the Antients*, is this, that when prepared, it will by an active Dissolution on other Concretes manifest their Medicinal Vertues; as, namely, on *Harts-horn*, *Unicorn's-horn*, *Crab's-eyes*, *Pearl* and *Coral*; it fixes *Mercury*, and dissolves all the Metals under *Sol* and *Lune*, from whence proceeds that variety of Specifick and Succedaneous Medicines, appropriated to Stubborn, Rebellious and Chronick Diseases, abundantly more than from the *Oleosum* it self, that being, in its Medicinal Vertue, only an Active, Dissolving and Abstersive Medicine, so passing the six Digestions, according to **Helmont**, unconquered, whose Specifick Vertue is to dissolve all the Tartarous Humours of the *Gout Preternatural Obstructions*, and the *Stone* or *Gravel* in the *Reins* or *Kidneys*

I have an Instance of this kind, as an undeniable Proof, in the Cure of a young Man, twenty Years of Age, in whom all Physitians allowed the Disease Hereditary, he being born with it; yet this same *Spirit* of *Tartar* would not cure an *Elephantiasis*, or *Pox*, but as it was specificated by *Mercury*, the only Specifick for those Diseases; neither would it hasten Delivery without the Appropriation of the

Liver

Liver of an Eel, Cinnamon or Unicorn's-horn, Specificks in that case; neither would it cure a Patient of mine, who was afflicted with a Fever, and given over as past hope; but as it was Specificated with the Sulphur of *Venus*, which Person is still alive to testify, that he was cured as with a Charm: Further, I tried the same upon another, who had an ill Habit of Body, Consumptive, and so far wasted, that Physitians said he was incurable; but it succeeded not, 'till Specificated with Oyl of Cinnamon, Myrrh, Aloes and Saffron, he was then restored thereby to a Miracle in less than a Month, *&c.*

From hence may easily be discerned the Ignorance of those, who pretend to cure all Chronick Diseases by one Medicine, and that but a slight and Volatile *Oleosum*, which will not pass beyond the Vessels of the second Digestion, and consequently only reaching acute Diseases: I do allow them to be pretty Medicines, but I would have them called by agreeable Names, the Field of Learning being large enough, without offering any Abuse to the Antients.

For the true Name and thing is only to be distinguished by the aforesaid Marks, which if it answers not, we may readily conclude the Authors as stupid, as the Apostate *Jews* of old, who said, the Fathers were fallen asleep, and all things remained as they were, and so regarded not the true *Messiah* when he came. With Divine Reverence to the Fountain, this I doubt is the State of our present

Oleosum-mungers, who think, that (the Antients being dead) there is no true Disciple remaining to essay their Proficiency, and therefore conclude, that their words may pass for current with the Ignorant, who are too easily imposed on.

But depend, that if your *Genuine Oleosum of the Antient Philosophers* (as you call it) will not bear the Probe, and that if you refuse to answer me the next Courant, I must count you an Impostor, Publishing to the World false Medicines in true Names, and that you are worthy to be exposed as such, for a Caution to the Ignorant, and an Information to the truly Ingenious, *&c.*

Observe Reader, tho' I sent to his House for an Answer to these, yet I received none; I suppose that Truth carried such a convincing Testimony with it, that he thought Silence the best way to stop my Mouth, or else, as some may imagine, that Silence is a Contempt, and that he would baffle me that way, which was not the Case here; for it wrought that Effect, that he alter'd his Advertisement in the Courant upon it, as may be easily proved, if the File of Courants is search'd, and therefore near about the same time I sent him this following Letter.

SIR,

SIR,

A Civil Anſwer to my Letter, ſeeing I wrote like a Son of Art, was but what was requiſite to have been perform'd on your part, as a pretended Brother; and your omiſſion in this has been the cauſe of theſe, and I cannot chooſe, but be plain to tell you, when I conſider your unadviſed Boldneſs in your Advertiſements and Book, eſpecially the two firſt Paragraphs, to ſo ſingle and ſlight a Medicine, ſeeing I am bold to aſſert, that *Human Urine* is the Subject of it, and that it is produced by an eaſie Artifice; for he that knows how to Concentrate new Urine, before it has taken any Ferments, and then Ferment by a ſecret Circulation, unites the two Salts, Volatile and fixed, with the ſecret Oleous Light, *viz.* That from whence the *Phoſphorus* proceeds; ſuch an one (I ſay, I am bold to tell you) needs not want the Wine of Urine, as good as yours; yours being not Homogeneous, nor a Spirit, as is demonſtrable by an eaſie Artifice, but ſeparable into two diſtinct Parts, which that which is Homogeneous can never be.

Therefore what you aſſert concerning its Name, and your Aſſurance thereon, ſaying, *'tis too evident to be confuted by the Artifice of any*; as alſo concerning its Preparation, when you ſay, *the Antients have left room for its Improvement to no ſmall Advantage of the Medicine*: And then wou'd inſinuate, that you

O 3 have

have brought it to such a Perfection, as not capable of an higher Exaltation, and that therefore it must consequently excel, and that not a little, what was prepared by old **Van Helmont.** All this I look upon such a piece of unparallel'd Cant and Banter, so great an Imposition upon the World, and Abuse to **Helmont,** that Morning Star of Art, that no Son of Wisdom can bear without Reproof; seeing you have vainly Arrogated to your self the Preheminency, and by a fond and foolish Conceit, make your self as much above him, as the Sun excels a Star; therefore it will be requisite to consider these things apart, and first of the Name.

As to the Name, I read not of any Urinous Spirits Entituled *Oleosums*, either in **Basil, Valentine, Paracelsus, Helmont** or **Starkey,** that being, I suppose, a newer Coin'd Word, taking its Rise from **Sylvius,** the *Famous Professor of* **Leyden**; nor do I read of any Medicines that deserve that Name but such as are included under these three Heads, *viz.* *Volatile Salt of Tartar*, *Liquor Alchahest*, and *Mercury of the Philosophers*, which are known by three distinct Marks, &c. the *Salt* of *Tartar* is a Saline Oily Medicine, the *Liquor Alchahest* an Oleous Saline Spirit, and the *Mercury* of *Philosophers* a Sulphureous Saline Butter: The first is made so by being Volatilized by Essential Oils and Vinous Spirits; the *Liquor Alchahest* is the Mercurial and Sulphureous Power united, by the forcible Dissolution of its own Body, and so brought into a Sa-

line

line Oil; and the Mercury of Philosophers is an Union of the Water, Blood and Spirit, the Body being dissolved by a Natural Process, which by a second Rotation becomes Duplicate; each of these bears a particular Mark or Character, by which it is to be known. The *Salt of Tartar* Oylified bears this Character, *sc.* its dissolving Vertue, as aforesaid, on Pearl, Crab's-eyes, and Unicorn's-horn, and all the Metals under *Sol* and *Lune*, and fixes *Mercury*. The *Liquor Alchahest* fixes *Mercury*, and dissolves all Bodies universally, yet it self remains Immortal. The *Mercury* of *Philosophers*, his Character is to dissolve Beings by way of Generation, but yours bearing none of these, by Consequence can't be the *Oleosum* of *the Antients*, nor that of **Helmont**, which he advanced to so great Perfection, as no Master breathing could ever exalt higher: His Mastership he has plainly shewn to the Sons of Wisdom by the Mechanick Proofs, *viz. Its dissolving a Charcole, fixing Mercury, so as to bear Test and Copel, and bringing Gold over the Helm*; therefore I think it the highest Arrogance in you, to pretend to amend that, which you know not any thing of: so that as yours deserves not the Name of an *Oleosum*, much less to be stiled the *Oleosum of the Antient Philosophers*.

For Secondly, The Nature of yours plainly shews that it deserves not the Name of *the Oleosum of the Antients*, nor indeed of an *Oleosum*, for an *Oleosum* is Globical and Fat, and being poured into Water, makes a Milky Fat-neſs there, by which a true *Oleoſum* may be known; but yours, not giving theſe Signs, in the leaſt, may be concluded not half a Medicine; for Urine is but the Recrement of Blood from the Nutriment taken in; the Blood is the Balſom, containing the Life, and Ferments, Lamp and Fewel of it; ſo that except the Eſſence of the Blood be therewith united, the Medicine is incompleat, and thoſe prepared from Urine alone are the meaneſt half, becauſe according to Helmont and others, from the Coagulating Urinous Spirits and Salts, the Gravel in the Reins and Kidneys, Joint and Chalky Gout have their Original, and my own Experience confirms the ſame, having twenty Years ago form'd Stones (like the *Duelech*) and Sand, in quantity, from Urinous Salts.

Thirdly, From what has been ſaid, the Nature and Inſufficiency of your Medicine may not only be diſcerned, but alſo your Deficiency in making good what you ſo publickly Aſſert; for Helmont was ſo compleat a Maſter, that he left no room for any Improvement, nor to excel in any degree whatever, what he prepared and enjoyed in his Time, and gave as an Hiſtory of in his Writings, concerning which that Worthy Son of Art, Philalethes bears his Teſtimony in theſe words, *That his Writings, when the World ſhould injoy them, would (be ſuppoſed) be the higheſt piece of Philoſophy that ever was written.* If I ſhould then ask you by what Authority you preſume to give Judgment concerning

ing his Attainments, I reckon you'll be highly baffled to give an anſwer, ſeeing your Age cannot demonſtrate that you were capable of any Knowledge of him by Acquaintance, yea, the moſt familiar Acquaintance in the World, ſo as to be converſant with him in his Operations; without which there could be no true Judgment of his Attainments: every Artiſt labouring in Chymiſtry, and enjoying Secrets, muſt aſſent to this Aſſertion; and if you ſhould ſay, you gather it from the Hiſtory of his Writings, that abſolutely requires Proof; for I can ſee no ſuch deficiency recorded there: And this Proof muſt not be Vaunting Cant, but demonſtrative, ſhewing the Nature of **Helmont's** Medicine, with which you parallel yours, and pretend to name it from, and wherein the Difficiency of **Helmont's** conſiſts; alſo the Nature of yours, and wherein you have excel'd, and when this is done I am well ſatisfied, the World will have very little Eſteem of your Medicine. But if you decline this, you have no room left to juſtifie your Proceedings, in ſpeaking ſo contemptiouſly of ſo great an Artiſt, and taking the Crown from off his Head, ſetting it on your own, as if to you belong'd the Maſterſhip, when all the while I am well ſatisfied, you are not worthy to hold him the Candle: May not we judge you of the number of thoſe, that ignorantly judge of things, they underſtand not, and ſhew that your deſign is but to baffle and banter the World, by putting great Names on Trivial

Medi

Medicines, imposing by false Glosses, to make your Market the greater.

I cannot pass by, without taking notice of another Absurdity, *viz.* your Assertion, *that the last Man on Record, that possessed this noble Medicine was Van* **Helmont**; but you are not pleas'd to cite that Record, whereby we might know what Name he call'd it, &c. If you would insinuate, as if it should be the *Alchahest*, you are in this Point also highly mistaken; for since him it has been possessed by the famous **Ludovicus de Comit**: by **Philalethes**, and some say by **Starkey**, as also the *Oleosum* of *Tartar* and *Urine*, but having written particularly concerning the latter, I shall now draw to a Conclusion; assuring you, that a Slight or Contempt shall not answer this, for seeing you have exposed a kind of Publick Challenge to the World in your Advertisements, I do expect that this shall have some Publick Answer, or else you may depend, I shall expose you to the Publick, and Print these Letters, of which, for that end I keep a Coppy, &c.

Thus, Reader, having given the Coppy of the Letters I sent to *Helmont*'s *Corrector*, I will leave the experienced, judicious, and unbyass'd to judge of it, and how far I have Truth and Verity on my side, and how far I am enabled by these Animadversions, and by daily Experience to vindicate so great a Master as **Helmont** was, whose Works Glory in their Author's Perfection and high Attainments, and most sound

Deli-

Deliveries; and as the *Volatile Salt of Tartar, and Liquor Alchabest* were enjoyed by him in their compleat and highest Perfection, and tho' he hath written of them in Ænigmatical Terms, because he would not have them too common, and hath given the Studious Opportunity to seek with indefatigable Labour, if ever he intend to obtain his desired end, yet it doth not follow that all who seek shall obtain; for as **Helmont** says, *God sells Art for Labour*, and 'tis infallibly so, in that the Knowledge of these things is the Gift of God, and all that run do not win the Prize; and the more the pitty we have but few *Pallases* in Art, to decide the Controversie, but the Golden Apple that was to be given to the fairest, was never by half so valuable to me as true Medicine, and such as carry a demonstrative Proof with them, and I never desire to attain an higher Perfection therein, than **Helmont** did in his days, and yet I might then value my self equal to the best Masters in *Europe*; so that there is no room to pretend the bettering of what **Helmont** has done, but on the contrary, all that do not understand him are by many thousand parts short of his Attainments, and the Scope that he has given in his Writings by only general Hints of the Preparation of his Medicaments, admits not of their being better'd; but the difficulty is, that many are thereby kept in *Dædalus*'s *Labyrinth* from obtaining; for that he is as difficult to be understood, as the

the Story of *Medea* and *Jason*, or the twelve Labours of *Hercules*, or any other of the Poetical and Philosophical *Ænigma's*, when they are obtained, they are known by the Signs and Demonstrations afore-given; so that those who pretend to be Masters of them without these Signs, I may say, they have long sung *Parturiunt Montes*, &c. So that I shall pass them by, and come to speak a few words concerning *Powers* and *Oleosums*, as an Introduction to the following Chapter.

Oleosums and *Powers*, wholly consist in an Union of their fixed Alchalizated Salts, Vinous Spirits, and Essential Oyls, after the same *Modus* as the Volatization of *Salt* of *Tartar*; therefore well might Starkey say, *the Prescription of these is rather a common place than single Receipt*, for if you learn one you learn all; and I have given you some candid Essays in the following Sheets, in order to the attaining thereof, but by the way I would have you to understand, that it is not so written, that every Hog may come to the Honey-pot. For where I speak of the most Interior sort, *viz.* Those prepared by *Sal-Armoniack*, you are not to understand the common *Sal-Armoniack*, for that will never effect it, but a Philosophical one, prepared wholly from the *General Spirit*, being Sulphureous, Fat and Bituminous, and has an internal, decocting Fire in it, which performs the Act of Union, superiour to the *Copavian Balm*, and is the very same, by which the *Salt* of *Tartar* is Vola-

Volatized; but these *Oleosums* and *Powers* are done in a short time by Cohobation, whereas the latter is done by secret Circulation and Decoction, and by length of time; nay, the Knowledge of this *Sal-Armoniack* is the very Key that opens the door to the obtaining of our *Sal Panaristos*; for without it you can never bring the Universal Elements to Harmony, and therefore has **Philaletes**, and other Adepts, call'd this *Sal Armoniack*, *Arsenicum*; for that the Philosophers *Arsenicum* is the flashing of Metals or their Salt, by which the other Principles are brought to Union and Durability, by a Natural Separation of their Impurities.

Reader, Meditate well on these Words, for they are worth thy time spent about them, and peradventure I have dropt that here, which may never more in so much plainness flow from my Pen, whilst I am on this side Eternity; in that I have at once given you the Key of all the Misteries that have been treated on since the Foundation of the World, and that the truly worthy may conceive so, as to enjoy, is the sincere Desires of your Cordial Friend.

CHAP.

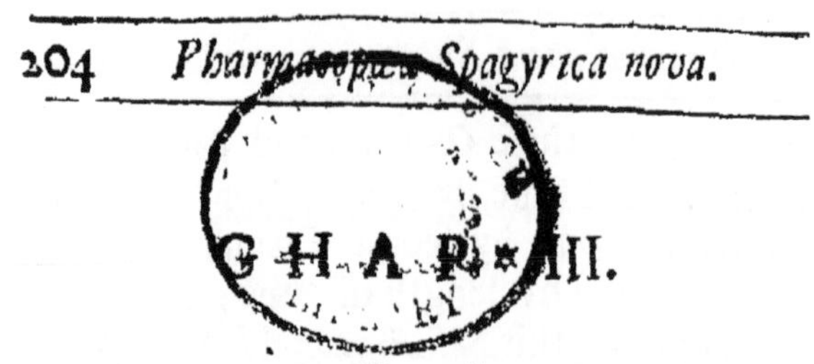

CHAP. III.

Potestates Nobilissimæ Succedaneæ & Specificæ per Sal : Tartari Volatil : or Noble Succedaneous Specifick Powers.

THE Foundation of these *Succedaneous Powers* is fixed *Alkalies*, produced by the Fire of Conflagration and Calcination from dried Herbs, as Mugwort, Wormwood, *&c.* Or from the *Argal* or Lees of Wine, which produces a noble Alkalie, no way inferior to any other whatsoever, and will supply the place of any of them, there being in *Tartar* whatever, may be said to be in any other fixed Salt; and therefore has **Starkey** not undeservedly named them *the Publick Family of Alkalies*, so that you need not be difficult in the choice of *Alkalies*, provided you have but that of *Tartar*; for you may work the same thing with it, as with the Salt of any other Vegetable, when united with their Essential Oils and burning Spirits, and will carry the same Tast, Vertue and Efficacy with it.

So that the great Business of Art, is to render the Salt Volatile, in order to obtain these *Succedaneous* and *Specifick Powers*: And here you are to observe, that what these Salts are deprived of in their being made fixed (for

(for that *Alkalies* are not a Product of Nature, but of Art) must be again added in a purified Degree for their Volatilization.

Now we see, that *Argal* parts with a more Volatile Urinous *Alkaly* in their Production, which is assumed by an Union of the more perfect Saline with the fixed and permanent Sulphur, and so becomes Alkalizate, and fixed with a kind of Metallick Fixation, so that we may readily conclude, that the Fury of *Vulcan* in this Act, does not only devour the Volatile Saline and Sulphurous Parts, we have been speaking of, but also their secret Tye of Life is sent away, together with that crude and undigested Air that violently fills the Pores of every Body, from whence comes the Dregs, Corruptions, Fætidness and Stink of all Oyls and Spirits; I speak this knowingly, like a Philosopher; for that this Crude Air or burning, fætid Sulphur being separated, the Principles become Balsamick and fragrant: We have an Example, what this Crude Air or Fæted Oil is, in the Oil of *Sea-coal*, *Soot*, *Hart's-horn*, and that of *Tartar*, which obtains not any kind of Sweetness, but by often Rectification, and that from some Mineral Earths, indued with an Acid Fixity to insorb these Corruptions.

Therefore what you deprive *Alkalies* of in their Fixation, must be again added in a purified Degree, for their Volatization, that is the Reason that *Essential Oils* and *Vinous Spirits*, if united by a due *Medium*, do again Volatilize them, but observe, this *Medium* must be not

not only Bituminous and Sulphureous, but also indued with that Tye of Life which they were deprived of in their Fixation, or else it will be impossible to bring the Principles again to Union

In the first place, therefore it is highly necessary that you know the Purification of *Salt* of *Tartar*, both from its Internal and External Foulness; the External is taken off by a Reiterate Dissolution and Congelation in Water; but the Internal only by a Fermentative Decoction, stirring up the Internal Fire, whereby the interwoven Attoms of Corruption and Defilements will be separated from the pure butterified Salt, which being brought to such a degree of Perfection, it is fitly prepared for its Volatilization, and Union with burning *Spirits* and *Essential Oils*; but these unite not, as I have already said, but by a proper *Medium*, which is bituminous and fat, of which there are two sorts, Particular and Universal; the Particular may be known by its Balmy Nature and Healing Qualities, and in Scripture it is described, where the Query is asked, *is there no Balm in Gilead? Is there no Physician there?* The Universal is a certain Volatile *Armoniack Salt*, of a middle Nature between *Mercury* and *Arsenick*, of a very fat and bituminous Nature, and universal Operation, as being the Bind and Tye of all the Elements, being also of a middle Nature, between a Body and a Spirit, and therefore called *Dispositio Media* I shall speak so much

con-

concerning these two *Mediums*, as I think convenient to make this Part compleat.

As to the first, the *Modus* is only to imbibe the *Salt* with this *Bituminous Matter*, first cleansed by Water in a moderate digestive Heat, as that of Hatching of Chickens, by a reiterated Operation, and hourly stirring, until it has made a full Ingress into the Body, and it becomes thereby so much satiated, that it refuses to take in any more; then you may Putrifie it in its own *Volatile Spirit*; and it will unite with it, and become Volatile, Spiritual and Transparent; which being distil'd over by *Cohobation*, *will then dissolve all green Vegetables, without heat in little time into their Essences and Powers, which will separate into two distinct Oils from all their Dead and Corrupt* Fæces: Let this suffice for the Particular.

As to the universal way, it is by uniting this said *General Medium* with the *Salt* of *Tartar*, in due proportion; and imbibe it with *Essential Oils*, until the Salt hath swallowed up enough to assatiate its Thirst, the which is called *Pondus Naturæ*; and this is performed by Humidations and Exsiccasions, or successive Feedings, and as the Worthy *Starkey* says, *they must be dried by the Air, and moisten'd by the Fire and Ferment of Nature*: So by a gentle Decoction brought to a total Volatility, and that in three Months time, according to Helmont, yet done without Water; for our Mercurial-Armoniack, and Universal Medium is first assatiated with his own Spirit or Vinegar, and so made Fat, Sulphureous and

Bituminous, containing an internal Fire of Union to Salts and Oils, and yet a Spiritual and Airy one for their Volatilization: These are the Air and Fire of Nature, and are the same Principles, tho' more crude, with those from whence the *Liquor Alkahest* does proceed; nay, there may proceed Matters or *Mediums* in your search for that Liquor, to wit, the *Alchahest*, (if upon a right Subject) which, tho' through your Errors, they are render'd unfit for that Work, yet may very well answer in the Volatilizing of *Tartar*, especially, such as are *Vinous* and of an *Armoniack* and *Bituminous Nature*, therefore, says the Worthy **Helmont**, *if you cannot obtain the Secret of our Fire, then learn to make the Salt of Tartar Volatile, and therewith perform your Dissolutions.*

The aforesaid *Essential Salts* are the true Foundation of the *Volatile* and *Genuine Spirit of the Antients*; and tho' these Salts do dissolve in Water, and mix without any Oiliness swimming on top, which shews their radical Union, they will again boil up without any loss of Vertue: But observe, the Water or Wine you dissolve them in, will, if distill'd, give in the first part a fragrant Spirit of a strong tast of the *Essential Oil* and *Salt*, yet that is not the true *Spirit* of *Tartar*; for if you stop your Operation, as the Flegm begins to come, and gently dry your *Salt* in a slow Fire of Nature, and then in the like Fire imbibe it with its own Spirit, till both become

one;

one, you may then mix that *Salt* with *Potters Earth*, and distil, and Cohobate till all is come over, which will then afford you good cause to Glory; in that you have obtain'd the *true* and *Genuine Spirit* of *Tartar*, of which Paracelsus, Helmont and Starkey so much boast; which performs all, both as to the dissolution of Concretes, and curing Diseases that they have ascribed to it.

But if these *Salts* are not dissolved in *Water* or *Wine*, but in the strong *Spirit* of *Wine*, or the highly *Rectified Spirit* of the Concrete, whether *Wormwood*, *Mint*, *Bawme*, *Cinnamon*, or the like, and their Spirits drawn off, part will ascend in a strong fragrant Spirit, which being saved till the Flegm comes, and then the Salt gently dried, as before, and imbibed with its own Spirit, till both become one, which they'll readily do; because you have that *Medium* that makes the fixed Salts, and them readily touch, and upon the bare touch, as *Helmont* says, *one third will be converted into Elementary Water*; which (I say) being gently dried becomes hungry, and must be fed with *Essential Oils* and *Vinous Spirits* so often, till they will sublime in the Form of a *Salt* in a gentle Fire, that being really necessary to preserve their Fragrancy, and then you have them in the highest degree of Perfection, that Art and Nature can advance them to.

By this Method you may obtain, not only the *Powers* of *Wormwood* and other Herbs, at a lower degree of Perfection, which I in my first Edition Published in Misterious Terms, under the Title of *Potestates Absynthii*; but alsoall sorts of *Essential Salts*, according to the Nature of the Oil you make them with: And 'tis observable in their Elixeration and Volatilization, the Oil will be wholly converted into a Chrystalline Salt, a small part only excepted, which will be turned into a Resinous Gum, distinct from what is Salified; which said Salt contains the *Vita Media* and whole *Crasis* of the Vegetable: For by this way of Union they contract from each other a wonderful Vertue; from the Salt proceeds the Abstersive, and from the Oil the Balsamick and Vital Nature, very fragrant, refreshing the Vital Spirits, and blotting out the *Diseasy Ideas*, as having pass'd thro' Death and Mortification, and are Regenerated from their fixed State to a new Life and Volatility, being of an Hermaphroditical Nature, retaining the Vertue of both Parents. These are those *Salts* so much commended by Van Helmont, who tells you, *that he who knows how to convert the Oil of Cinnamon, by means of its own Alkaly into a Saline Nature, has a certain Cure for the Apoplexy and Palsie*, and in another place, *that the Salt of Wormwood, thus made, is a true Specifick for the Cure of all kind of Fevers.*

Here is a large Field for Medicine, for if you learn to make one *Essential Salt*, you learn all, so that you may at pleasure make great variety, as of *Cloves*, *Mace*, *Nutmegs*, *Fennel*, *Cummin*, *Coriander*, *Orange*, *Juniper*, *Rosemary*, *Camomile*, and the like; nay, even of of things Gummous, as *Turpentine*, *Amber*. 'Tis obſervable that theſe Salts in ſhooting take on the Form of Sugar-candy.

Obſerve, by the ſame Rule alſo is obtained the *Balſam Samech* of **Helmont** and **Paracelſus**, which is only an Union of pure *Salt* of *Tartar* with pure *Spirit* of *Wine*, digeſted and brought to a Balſam, which ſome about Town have been pretending to finiſh theſe twenty Years; and I will give 'em Twenty more, eſpecially one of 'em, who I am well ſatisfied is abundantly ignorant of the *Univerſal Medium*, by which it is performed, and yet uſes the freedom to call others *Jumblers in Chymiſtry*.

This *Samech* may be united with the Corrected Tincture of any Vegitable, eſpecially of *Opium*, and you've a certain Cure for a Troop of Diſeaſes; or you may make it Saline, and then unite it with the Macerated Tincture of any Vegetable; for theſe Salts have a Communicative Ferment to them; then digeſt in a Chicken-heat, and 'twill all in about twelve or fifteen Days be converted into a Chryſtalline Salt.

Thus, the *Tincture* of *Wormwood* exalts its own *Salt*, and ſo the like of other Vegetables: Nay, moreover, you may by this way have a *Salt* of ſuch Herbs, as will not by Diſtillation yield their *Eſſential Oils*, as of *Hellebore*, *Jallop*, *Briony*, *Elecampane*, and many others, nay, even from *Saffron*, and many things of a more Gummous Nature. By this means you may, through Cohobation with the *Eſ-*

ſential Oil, bring over the *Sulphur* of any of the inferiour Metals and Minerals, even of *Sulphur Vive*, in the form of a *fœtid* Oyl, which being ſeparated from all its Flegm, and Elixerated, and made fragrant with Aromatick Spirits, as *Cardamum*, *Cinnamon*, and the like, then brought to an *Eſſential Salt* or *Samech*, you have a Medicine, on which you may rely in the moſt difficult Caſes.

In your Elixerations and Volatizations you may make a Compound of *Eſſential Oils* and *Tinctures*, according to their Specifick Vertues, appropriated to Diſeaſes; for Example, I will give you two or three which I approve of.

For the Diſeaſes of the Head, In the firſt place, I approve of the Compoſition of the *Apoplectick Balſam*, which is as follows, ℞ *Oyl of Nutmegs by expreſſion* ℥ii, *Oil of Cloves*, *gutt.* 20, *Oils of Mace*, *Lavender*, *Sweet-marjoram Cinnamon*, *Rhody*, *ana. gutt.* 15. *Balſam of Peru*, *enough to incorporate them in a Marble Mortar to a Balſam*, *then add Maſtick*, *Civet*, *Ambergreece*, *ana. gutt* 6

Let theſe be Elixerated with Oil of *Roſemary*, and brought into a *Samech* with the Tincture of *Lavender*, *Roſemary flowers*, and *Roſa Solis*.

For the Diſeaſes of the Breaſt and Stomach, you may Elixerate with Oil of *Cinnamon*, *Turpentine*, and white Oil of *Amber*, together with the Oil of *Bawm*; and bring into a *Samech* with the Tincture of *Coral*, or of *Liquorice*, *Elecampane*, *Gentian*, *Galingal*

Galingal taken out in the ſtrong Spirit of *Scurvy-graſs.*

For Wind, Gripes and Chollick, Elixerate your *Salt* of *Tartar* with oil of *Aniſeeds,* and Chymical oil of *Camomile flowers,* and bring it to a *Samech* with the Tincture of *Opium, Myrrh, Aloes* and *Saffron,* and then you've a Medicine for the Cure of twenty other Diſeaſes.

For the Stone, Elixerate your *Salt* with oil of *Turpentine,* and the white oil of *Gum Animi,* and bring it into a *Samech* with the Tincture of *Arſmart, Cinnamon* and *Opium.*

For the Pox, Scurvey and **Leprosie,** and **Virulent Gonorrhæa's,** Elixerate your *Salt* with oil of *Saſſafraſs,* and the white oil of *Soot,* and bring it to a *Samech* with the Tincture of *Gum Guaiacum,* and *Balſam Capavii* and *Sarſaparilla.*

Now in the Elixeration, if you add the *Sulphur* of *Antimony, Venus* or *Spelter,* and then diſtil into a Volatile Spirit, by Cohobation, as before directed, and Cohobate on *Common Mercury,* 'till it comes to a middle Fixation, you will have a Medicine, in which you may Glory, for the Cure, not only of the foreſaid Diſeaſes, but alſo of all other Refractory ones whatever.

For **Asthmaes, Consumptions, Palsies, Apoplexies, inveterate Vertigoes,** or **Swimmings in the Head,** Elixerate your *Salt* with oil of *Cinnamon, Cloves,* and *Cedar*; and bring it into a *Samech* with the Tincture of *Cedar* and *Bawm*; digeſt 'till it

Salifies, and is brought to a Volatility and fragrant Nature; then have you a Medicine that will perform all, what can be expected from a Vegetable Remedy, and does very much contribute to long Life. The Medicines thus prepared, are not undeservedly called *Alkalium Apex*, or the top of Alkalies, and Crown of the Physician. *The Dose* not *exceeding* 15 *or* 20 *Grains at most.*

From what has been said, you may see there is an Affinity between *Essential Oils*, *Vegetable Tinctures* and *Vinous Spirits*, as also in the way of Working, between the Elixeration with Essential Oils, and bringing it to a *Smech* with *Spirit* of *Wine*: But in the end there is this difference, the one Distils in the Nature of a *Spirit*, and the other Sublimes in Form of a *Salt*.

Now that you may not be to seek of Appropriated *Specificks*, some not being satisfied without a large Field, I'll give you a small Table, Collected above twenty Years ago, as follows.

For the Diseases of the Head, the *Sulphur* of *the Vitriol* of *Venus*, and of *Lune* and *Mercury*, or any precious Stones wrought up with *Oil of Rosemary*, *Lavender* and *Cinnamon*, and the *Tinctures* of *black* and *white Hellebore* and *Opium*, and then Aromatized with the *Spirit* of *Coriander-seeds*, *Cardamums*, and *Cinnamon*; this is also an excellent *Splenetick*. Or thus, *Hellebore*, *Asarum*, *Briony-roots* and *Jallop*, sometimes that and *Opium*, which is then called *Elixir Laudan Cephalicum & Splenetricum*, or or an Easer of Pain, appropriated to the Head and Spleen.

For the Diseases of the Thorax or Breast, I approve of *Opium*, *Pearl*, *White Talk*, and the *Sulphur* of *Lead*, wrought up with *Oil* of *Cedar*, *Oleum Regeneratum*, and the fixed Oil of the *Fir-tree*, Oil of *Oranges*, *Fennel* and *Lillies*, with the Tincture of *Saffron*, *Mary-gold-flowers*, *Radishes*, *Lignum Aloes*, and *Pepper*; and then Aromatized with *Spirit* of *Caraway-seeds*, *Cummin-seeds*, *Nutmegs*, *Cardamums* and *Coriander-seeds*.

For the Diseases of the Stomach, the *Sulphur* of *Juniper*, and of the *Metallus Masculus* is very good, with the *Oil* of *Bawm*, *Pepper*, *Wormwood* and *Citron-peels*, being brought into a *Samech* with the *Tincture* of *Gentian*. *Scordium*, *Hellebore*, *Rhubarb*, *Raisins* and *Cassia*, and then Aromatized with Spirit of *Bawm*, *Angelica*, *Saffron*, *Rosemary-flowers*, *Cochenele* and *Cinnamon*.

For the Diseases of the Intestines and Guts, the *Sulphur* of *Mars*, or *Venus* is very proper; with the *Oil* of *Bay-berries*, *Juniper-berries*, *Cinnamon* and *Camomile-flowers*, brought into a *Samech* with *Tincture* of *Opium*, *Pilewort*, *Myrtle*, *Sumach*, *Betony*, *Satyrion* and *Camphore*; *Aromatized* with Spirit of Sweet *Fennel-seeds*, *Cinnamon*, *Cloves* and *Mace*: But for Fluxes, you may use *Storax*, *Caranna*, *Gum Gutta*, which is also good for Coughs; but for violent Costiveness, temper with *Colloquintida*, *Aloes* and *Balsam* of *Peru*.

For

For the Diseases of the Liver, use *Antimony*, made into a *Regulus*, and its *Sulphur* separated, or the *Sulphur* of *Mercury*; Elixerate with *Oil* of *Tar*, *Lignum Rhodium*, and *Guaiacum*, and bring into a *Samech* with *Tincture* of *Elecampane-roots*, *Rhubarb* and *Horse-radish*, Aromatizing with *Spirit* of *Cinnamon* and *Lign. Cassia*.

For the Diseases of the Spleen, take the *Sulphur* of *Saturn*, and Elixerate with *Oil* of *Amber*, *Turpentine*, and *Juniper*, and bring into a *Samech* with *Tincture* of *Spleenwort*, *Satyrion*, *Black Hellebore*, *Calamint*, *Cortex Jesuiticum*, *Snake-root*, *Palma Christi*, and then Aromatize with *Spirit* of *Bawm*, *Mint*, *Rosemary-flowers*, and *Coriander seeds*; this is also excellent for the Cure of Agues, *&c.*

For Diseases of the Lungs, and Mesentery or sweet Bread, take the *Sulphur* of *Juniper*, or *Talk*, resolved, and Elixerate with Oil of *Bawm*, *Oleum Regeneratum*, and *Oil* of *Myrtles*, and conform into a *Samech* with *Tincture* of *Opium*, *Angelica*, *Spanish Zedory*; and in the time of the Plague add the Tincture of *Contrayerva*, *Scorzonera*, *Vincitoxicum*, *Snake-root* and *Burdock*, then to Aromatize it, make use of *Aqua Pestilentia*, as prescribed in our *Chymicus Rationalis*.

For the Diseases of the Reins, take *Sulphur* of *Vitriol*, or *Sulphur Universale*, and Elixerate with *Oil* of *Turpentine*, *Aniseeds* and *Juniper*, and for Tincture use that of *Saxifrage* *Galengale* *Marsh-mallows*, the *Cyprus-tree*, and *Buck-thorn-berries*, the Juice being brought to

a

a Rope, and then the Tincture taken; and for an Aromatick, the Spirit of *Corianders* and *Allspice*.

Observe, the Artist is no way confin'd to these Prescriptions, but may vary them himself, according as Reason shall best guide him, only remembring that he always take such Appropriated *Specificks*, as are of the most general Tendency; that so a few Medicines may cure a great many Diseases; for I am one of them that esteem not a multitude of Medicines, but rather covet to reduce Practice to six or seven.

When you are Master of the *Essential Salts*, you may obtain very good Medicines, without exalting them to the highest degree of Perfection; for these *Essential Salts* will in highly *Rectified Spirit* of *Wine*, again admit of the corrected Tincture of the Vegetables to be Extracted; for if you put *Spirit* of *Wine* on these *Essential Salts*, and then digest in a gentle Heat, the *Spirit*, by refusion or pouring off, as often as it is Tinged, will Extract the whole *Tincture* of the Vegetables, leaving the *Salt* behind robb'd of the same: From whence it may be gather'd that the *Salt* and *Tincture* are Centrally distinct, tho' they have Centrally wrought each on the other: Then this *Spirit* of *Wine* being distill'd off in a gentle Heat, the *Tincture* will remain, and is the whole *Crasis* of the Concrete; which is a noble Preparation for such Concretes as are Balsamick and Odoriferous, and where the Tincture is desired free from the mixture of

Salts

Salts, as namely, where the bare Refresh-ment without Abstersion is desired and required.

Thus is made the most noble *Aroph* of Helmont out of *Satyrion*, and may be used, either the *Tincture* alone, separated from the *Salt* by Extraction with *Spirit* of *Wine*, or mixed with the *Elixerated Salt*; which I rather approve and choose, unless in case, where the Back is to be strengthen'd, as in Women afflicted with Wasting; otherwise the Abstersiveness of the Saline Elixir promotes the Cure of the *Nephritis*, and *Stone* or *Gravel*.

By this way of Working you may command a *Salt* from *Opium*, which is a wonderful *Arcanum* for *Fevers*, *Agues*, and *Tormenting Pains*, the like from *Hellebore* for *Melancholy*, *Madness* and *lingring Fevers*. Thus, knowing these *Salts*, you have a true Key whereby you may command Nature's choicest Specifick Medicines, which are shut up in the most virulent and poisonous Vegetables, as also their pure Sulphurs, in which the Form and Light of every Being inhabits; which Light is their Life, and in it self is of a Saline, Transparent and Chrystalline Nature, and contains the whole Vertue of that Being, whence Extracted, for Light has a general Tendency, of which there be two sorts, Universal and Particular: The Universal had no other Birth but Manifestation; for in the Separation of the *Chaos*, it took its place in the superior Waters to illuminate inferior Beings: The Particular is some Portion of

Rays

Rays of the Universal, Concreted and Specificated by the Finger of God in every Texture, by which it is upheld, as the Band and Tye of their Form in all Generation: But seeing so small a quantity is sufficient for the life of every Concrete, it inhabits a large *Domicil* of Corruptions; therefore is the Extracting it apart very difficult, but being Extracted it very manifestly displays its Vertues, in chasing or driving away darksome *Ideas*; which are the Original and Procatartick Cause of Diseases; and this it performs by aiding and assisting the Vital Flame in us, which the diseasie Power and dark *Idea* labours to obnubilate, suppress and vanquish; so that the Central Life, mustering up its Forces, in order to preserve it self from this insulting Enemy, is by every Action or Flash debilitated; insomuch, that without a proper help, to wit, true Medicine, Nature still grows weaker and weaker, the Disease prevails, and the Lamp of Life is at length extinguished.

This being sufficient for general Rules, and as an Introductive Key to open the Treasury of *Specifick Medicines*, I shall now proceed to more particular Applications of *Select Specificks*, that so the Ingenious may not be defective in the true Art of Healing, *&c.*

CHAP.

CHAP. IV.

The Preparation of Specifick Powers *by the* Medium *of the* Volatile Salt *of* Tartar.

Being a further Illustration of the former Chapter.

IN this Chapter, I shall now come to shew the Preparation of *Specifick Powers*, which are Succedaneous to nothing but the Grand *Arcanums*, so much Gloried in by the Worthy *Starkey*, and the thrice Renowned *Helmont*, the Chymical Monarch, *Paracelsus*, and the Reverend and Learned *Basilius Valentinus*, and first of,

Potestates Cochleariæ, *or, Powers of Scurvy-grass.*

Take three or four Bushels of *Scurvy-grass* about the latter end of *May*, or beginning of *June*, stamp it, and add a peck of *Sugar-bakers-lime*, or others, which being distil'd will give you about two Gallons of Spirit; but be sure as soon as ever it comes weak to change the Receiver, for it will be ill tasted: With this Spirit moisten as much stamped *Scurvy-grass* as it will, and then add a Gallon of *Treacle*

cle, and bring it into the highest Fermentation, and distill into *Low-wines*; and after that by Addition of fresh *Scurvy-grass* into *Proof-goods*, and lastly into *Ætherial Spirits*: Which being thus prepared, are the most Fragrant and Vital of any other; the Grass has its chief Vertue in a Volatile Salt, and so having very little *Essential Oil*, or *fixed Salt*, the *Powers* are very difficult to be made; but to supply this Defect, I use the following *Oil* and *Salt* of *Tartar*.

Take three or four Bushels of *Scurvy-grass*, bruise it, *Mustard seed* half a Bushel, *Horse-radish* a Peck sliced; ferment forty eight hours with Water and Salt, in a Vessel close cover'd with Cloaths; then distil your *Essentitial Oil*, separate from the Water, and let the Water serve for new beginnings.

Then take pure *Salt* of *Tartar* half a pound, Elixerate and Unite with the foresaid *Essential Oil* by the aforesaid *Medium*, and so long with the *Oil* and *Spirit* feed it until it comes to a *Chrystalline Salt*; of this *Salt* add four ounces to every quart of your *Ætherial Spirit*, digest nine days in a gentle Heat, and so is your Powers prepared.

These are Succedaneous to nothing in the Scurvy, Jaundice, Dropsie, consumption, Shortness of Breath, and the like. Dose, from one drop to ten or fifteen in a Glass of fragrant Wine.

Pote-

Poteſtates Sambuci, *The Powers of Elder.*

Let the *Berry*, when fully ripe be gathered in its right Signature, and the Juice preſſed forth from the Husk (becauſe as we have ſaid in our *First Part*, in thoſe lies the Violent, Narcotick and Intoxicating Quality) Ferment, and work up with *Molaſſes*, as in other *Powers*; bring them into *Low-wines*, and then Rectifie from the *Flowers* into *Proof-goods*, and laſtly exalt it into *Æthereal Spirits*. Then let the white oil of *Amber* be often rectified from *Dwarf-elder*, till it becomes very fine; then take pure *Salt* of *Tartar*, Elixerate and Unite with this *Oil* by the *Medium* aforeſaid, and bring it to a *Chriſtalline Salt*; to which add your *Æthereal Spirit*, as in the laſt, digeſt and unite.

Theſe are very prevalent in Surfeits, Fevers and Small-pox, Dropſie, Scurvy and Hypocondriack Melancholly, Stone and Gravel: The Doſe from five to twenty drops in good Rheniſh Wine.

Poteſtates Roſmarini, *The Powers of Roſemary.*

Theſe are made as the former, the Herb being firſt Fermented and brought into *Low-wines*, then rectified from the *Flower* into *Proof-goods*, and ſo exalted into *Ætherial Spirits*;

Spirits: Then take *Rosemary-tops* and *Flowers*, what quantity you please, stamp them, and put them into a Glass, adding thereto warm Water, or rather Wine, with a little *Bay-salt*, stop it very close, and set it in a warm place ten days, then distil in a Sand-heat with a soft Fire, and you'll have an Oil and Water, which separate. *Rosemary* will afford you *Salt* enough for your Work, therefore take what quantity you please, burn it in a Fire of Conflagration, and from the Ashes extract a *Salt*, which Elixerate with its own *Essential Oil*, and bring it into a *Chrystalline Salt*, which being joined with your *Ætherial Spirit*, digest and unite, as aforesaid.

As its Vertues are many, so are they superior, especially for strengthning the Head, Memory and Sight; it comforts the Nervous Juices, and fortifies Nature against many Diseases. The Dose is from five to fifteen drops in fragrant Wine. This for cleansing and imbellishing the Complexion, abundantly surpasses the Hungarian *Water, bearing away the Garland from all common Preparations of Rosemary whatever.*

Potestates Absynthii, *Powers of Wormwood.*

Take of *Wormwood* (gathered in its Prime, to wit, in the latter end of *July*, or the beginning of *August*) Ferment and bring it into *Low-wines*; rectifie from fresh *Wormwood* into *Proof-goods*, and *Ætherial Spirits*: Then take a large quantity of *Wormwood*, chop it ſmall, and put it into a Tub, cover it with Water two or three Fingers, adding two or three handfuls of *Bay-ſalt*; ſo let it Ferment (as in other *Powers*) then diſtil therefrom the *Eſſential Oil*; remove and ſeparate by a Separatory, and carefully preſerve the *Oil*: The Water will ſerve to macerate freſh *Wormwood*, to which, being put into the Still, you may add the former Oil, and diſtil again by which means you will not only get the larger quantity of oil, but the ſame will alſo be purer and richer of the *Eſſential Vertues* of the Herb Now for the *Salt*, take a large quantity of the dried *Wormwood*, burn it to Aſhes in a Chimney, which put into a large *Hippocrates*'s *Sleeve*, hanging over a large Funnel, where is placed a double cap Paper, then gently pour upon the Aſhes diſtill'd Rain water about Blood-warm, which, diſſolving the Salt, will paſs through the Bag, and be received by the Funnel, from thence filtering into the under Receiver, will become very pure: You muſt obſerve to caſt on freſh Liquor as long as any Saltneſs comes out of the Aſhes, and when they will give no more, place your Receiver in a Sand-furnace, give Fire, and continue the ſame till the whole is Evaporated to a drineſs; then remove and put it into a Calcining Pot in a Wind-furnace, and with a ſmall Iron-rod keep ſtirring until it is throughly glowing hot; then take out, and when cold put them on a Marble or Glaſs, made for that purpoſe; ſet in a cold Cellar,

and

and let run *per deliq.* the which again Filter and Chryſtallize and then you have the true *Salt* of *Wormwood*, which ſome ſo much commend for *ſtopping Vomitings.* But to obtain the ture *Eſſential Salt*, wherein the Vertue of the *Wormwood* conſiſts, Spagyrically unite the *fixed Salt* with its *Eſſential Oil*, by our *Diſpoſitio Media*, which is the *Reconciler* of *Extreams*, and by a ſlow Fire, like the heat of the Sun in *Aries*, let it be nouriſhed till it Chryſtallizes; unite theſe Chryſtals with the *Æthereal Spirit*, ſo are your *Powers* prepared.

This moſt noble Medicine is not only a true Specifick in all kind of Fevers, but alſo cleanſeth and ſtrengthens the Stomach, removes Obſtructions of the Liver, and cleanſes by Urine, it ſtops Vomiting, even of Blood, cures the Tympany, expels Worms, reſiſts Putrifaction, and infallibly cures a ſtinking Breath; the Salt laid among Cloaths preſerves from Moths and Gnats. The Doſe of theſe Powers is from one to ten drops, in what Wine you pleaſe.

Poteſtates Roſarum, *The Powers of Roſes.*

Take *Roſe-leaves* one Buſhel, and Ferment with their own cold diſtilled Water, by the Addition of *Hony*, and diſtil into *Low-wines*; then rectifie from freſh Leaves into *Proof-goods* and *Æthereal Spirits.* Then take Roſe-leaves and moiſten with their own cold diſtill'd Water, adding to every pound of the Leaves *Sugar-candy* and decripitated *Bay-ſalt*, of each an ounce, *Cream* half a pint; putrifie in a warm place for the ſpace of three Months, then diſtil according to Art, and ſeparate the Oil from the Water, which reſerve for new beginnings: Then, ſeeing you can obtain no Salt, but from the Roſe-trees burnt; therefore to ſupply the Defect, make uſe of the *Butterrified Salt* of *Tartar*, the which Elixerate with the *Eſſential Oil*, and by a digeſtive Heat, nouriſh and bring to a *Chryſtalline Salt*, which being united with the *Ætherial Spirit*, the *Powers* are compleat.

Which are moſt powerful in all Dejections of the Mind, prevalent againſt Sounding Fits, Vertigoe, and Suffocation in Women; it eaſes all Pains of the Head, by anointing the Temples therewith: It revives all the Spirits, Natural, Vital and Animal, and therefore a great preſervative againſt all Peſtilential and Contagious Diſeaſes: In the Elevation you may mix it with Oil of Rhodium, Cloves and Oranges, and then you have a Medicine little inferior to an Aurum Potabile: The Doſe of theſe is from five to twenty drops, theſe are alſo of great Service for bathing of Inflamations, Gangrenes, &c.

Poteſtates Paragoricæ, *the Bathing Powers.*

Take *Roſemary-flowers*, *Lavender-flowers*, *Bawm*, *Mint*, and *Spaniſh Angelica*, of each a like quantity, Ferment with *Molaſſes*, and diſtil into *Low-wines*, and then with *freſh Flowers*, &c. Rectifie into *Proof-goods* and *Ætherial*

Spirits;

Spirits: Then Elixerate the *Salt* of *Tartar* with the *Essential Oils* of the abovesaid, and by the foregoing Process exalt to a *Chrystalline Salt*, which being united with the *Ætherial Spirit* the *Powers* are at hand.

Then take of these one pound, *Powers* of *Roses* four ounces, *Capurnian Bittumen* two ounces, dissolve and unite, and so it is prepared.

'Tis most excellent for bathing any grieved Part, and for mitgating any Pain in the Head and Teeth; diverting the Rheum from sore Eyes; 'tis also good in Bruises, Squats and Inflamations, also inwardly 'tis excellent for Fluxes, resisting Putrifaction, and therefore good in Pestilential Times. The Dose inwardly from four to twelve drops. 'Tis also an excellent Fucus to Beautify the Skin.

Potestates Hordei, *an Ensensificated Aqua Vitæ.*

Take a Barrel of Stout Brew'd Beer, rich and mellow, and half a Bushel of fresh Malt, distil into *Low-wines*; Rectifie from good Malt into *Proof-goods*, and after that into *high Spirits*; save all your Wash, and drain off all the clear from the *Faces*; heat the clear, and mash therewith on fresh Malt, and make a very strong Elixerated Wort, precipitate your Wort immediately with *Salt* of *Tartar*, and gently bring it to the Consistence of Hony, and take out the Tincture with its own

Spirit, as long as any is to be taken, with which Elixerate half a pound of the *Salt* of *Tartar*, working them by the *Universal Medium*, in all things, as you do the *Balsam Samech*, and feed to the utmost height which Art can bring them to; and then being diffused in its own *high Spirit* you have the true *Powers*.

These Powers are a perfect Balm in Nature, they resist Putrifaction, quench Thirst, and abate Fevers, and are indued with a Preservative Vertue, both to the Body of Man and Liquors: If they are prepared by a gentle Fire, and their Fragrancy well retained and advanced, an ounce of them being put into a Barrel of Beer will preserve it an Age in its Pristine Vigour and Pallatable Goodness yet indue it with all their Medicinal Vertues.

Potestates Vini, *the Powers of Wine.*

Take a Hogshead of good generous Wine, distil into *Low-wines*, *Proof goods*, and *Æthereal Spirits*; dry the *Faces*, and in a *Glaubers Furnace* distil them into *Oil*, and *Spirit*, which *Oil* Rectifie till it is white and fragrant, Calcine the *Salt*, extract and dry it, then Calcine again and shoot it into Chrystals very clear; which then Assatiate with the true *Spirit* of *Wine Vinegar*, which a considerable quantity will but serve to perform, then distil in a *Glaubers Furnace*, and you'll have an *Oil* and *Spirit*, which *Oil* also Rectifie till white and fra-

fragrant, and then it is that which I call *Oleum Tartari Regeneratum*, Calcine the *Caput Mort*, and extract the *Salt*, and purifie, as before; Elixerate your *Salt* with these two *Oils*, and in digestive Heat, by a proper *Medium*, Unite and Chrystallize, which then being again diffused in the *Æthereal Spirit*, your Powers are compleat.

Whose Vertues are General, Powerful in the Cure of Dropsie, Scurvy, Stone and Gout, being a great Secret, and Noble Specifick in the Cure, and preserving of Wines, as those of Malt are for Beer.

Potestates Prophelacticæ Imperiales.

* Take an Hogshead of the best *Canary*, *Flowers* of *Rosemary* and *Elder*, *Sweet-marjoram*, *Bawm*, *Brooklime*, *Scurvy-grass*, *Water-cresces*, *Mugwort*, *Clary*, *Arsmart*, *Mustard*, *Daucus* and *Horse-radish*, of each four pound; distil into *Low-wines*, which I call *Vinum Assatum*; and to make the *Vinum Fortificatum*, take *Lavender-flowers*, *Rosemary-flowers*, Flowers of the *Lilly of the Valley*, *Rosa Solis*, *Cowslip-flowers*, *Orange-flowers* (or for want of them the dry Pill) *Sage*, *Betony*, *Bugloss*, *Mint*, *Bawm*, *Angelica*, *Bay-leaves*, of each two pound, and distil into *Proof-goods*; then take *Citron-seeds*, *Peony-seeds*, *Cinnamon*, *Nutmegs*, *Cardamums*, *Sassafrass*, *Cubebs*, *Yellow-saunders*, *Lignum Aloes*, *Jujubes*, new, good and stoned, of each half a pound, all being Pul-

verized and Macerated, diſtill into *Aireal Spirits*; then take *Salt* of *Tartar* half a pound, Oil of *Roſemary*, *Saſſafraſs*, *Cinnamon*, *Juniper* and *Oleum Regeneratum*, of each a like quantity; Eliverate and bring into an *Eſſential Salt*, as in other Preſcriptions, and then unite the *Salt* and *Aireal Spirits*, ſo have you theſe *Powers* at command.

This highly exalted Cordial Medicine, or **Family Drops**, *which I formerly called the* **Travellers Companion**, *is a noble Antipeſtilential, Sudorifick Epileptick and Antipeleptick, of Health promoting Vertues, being a powerful Specifick againſt moſt Diſeaſes that may too ſuddenly approach, either by Repletion or Inanition, preventing the Spirits and animal Life from being ſeized by Poiſon or Poiſonous Vapours: It likewiſe ſtrengthens the Languiſhing Fountain of Life, and reſtores drooping Spirits, being ſo highly impregnated with the Oily Fuel of Light, as to be endued with ſuch reſtorative Vertues, that 'tis proper for all Ages, Sexes and Conſtitutions, let the Diſeaſe proceed from what Cauſe or Cauſes ſoever: For if you will but obſerve the Compoſition and Preparation, with the Specifick Vertue, you'll not think it ſtrange to be call'ed Imperial: This Medicine is much exalted by the Balſamick Ens of Tartar, whence it fails not of being a true Friend to the Diſeaſed, and is prevalent againſt the Lethargy, Palſie, Apoplexy, Epilepſie, Convulſion, Megrim and Calenture; 'tis alſo powerful againſt thoſe Diſeaſes of the Thorax, as Aſthma's, Pluriſies, ſpitting of Blood, Conſumption, Syncope,*

cope, Palpitations, &c. *Taking off the original Cause in Surfeits, whether they come through ill Cookery and unsavory Food, Excess in Eating or Drinking, or are occasion'd by long Fasting, Watching, or immoderate sleeping on the Earth; for the Motion of the Body being still, the evil Vapour is received, which dulls the vital Spirits, and contracts Diseases; nay, in fine, causes an Hydropical Humour, which banes and causes Men to dye like rotten Sheep; as is often experienced in Camps and Armies, as also in the* West-Indies.

Now this fortifies Nature against Assaults, and therefore prevalent against sudden Fears and great Surprizals; and when a diseasie Idea is introduced, this wonderfully appeases the Fury of the inraged Archæus, setling the Spirits in due decorum; 'tis also prevalent against the Diseases of the Intestines, Spleen, Pancreas, &c. *As the Cholick, Iliack Passion, Lientery, Diarrhœa,* &c, *Also against Agues, Plague, Measles and Small-pox, with other such Diseases, whether Infectious or Pestilential, as may be found, if but timely used, 'tis a true Specifick, either to imbibe or drive forth the original Cause of Diseases from the Center, for it works principally by Sweat, Urine and insensible Transpiration: 'Tis prevalent also against the Suffocations of the Womb, Obstructions,* &c. *Fortifying the Female Sex with Strength and vigorous Activity; 'tis also excellent against Weariness and Numbness of the Limbs, Bruises, Squats, Sprains and Cramps; for it disperseth and dissipates the Humour, and dissolves coagulated Blood, whether it comes from an internal Cause, or external Accident*: *This supplies the Defect of most simple Spirits, and indeed many of the other Powers.*

Let Travellers, whether by Sea or Land, and those that are subject to the foresaid Diseases, never be without a bottle of it, and in sudden Swoonings, Faintings, Apoplexies, or Convulsions, let them pour out some of it upon the Palm *of their Hand, and rubbing their Hands together, clap them to their Nostrils that the Savours may ascend, also strike their Temples and fore-part of their Head, and Chords of the Neck therewith; let this be often repeated, and if the Paroxism be strong, then take inwardly fifteen or twenty drops in Water or Wine.*

This is a great Preservative against the Plague, and other infectious Fumes, for which take ten or twelve drops in a glass of Water or Wine, or other proper Vehicle, and repeat it three times a day, and dipping the end of an Handkerchief therein, rub your Nostrils therewith: This Method is to be observed in Surfeits, *Measles,* Small-pox, *or* Swine-pox, *and many other acute Diseases, and where it is too strong for weak Natures to be taken in Wine, let it be drank in Bawm or Rosemary Posset-drink, and promote Sweating thereon.*

For the Gripes of the Guts, Strangury and difficulty in making Water, it must be drank in its largest Dose in Rhenish-wine, or rather in the distill'd Water of Arsmart. For Rickets in Children, it must be applied as well outwardly as inwardly, chafing the grieved part therewith before

the

the Fire, and dipping a Scarlet Cloth therein, laying it on the part afflicted: This repeat as often as occasion requires, and swath from the Armpits to the Groins with a Linnen Swath; which Method is well to be observed for weak and pained Limbs.

By these Examples you may compose what sort of *Powers* you please; for if you understand the Mistery of our *Philosophical Medium* and *Spirit* of *Wine*, these Misteries cannot be hid from you: Therefore what I have written here, being sufficient for this Head, I shall proceed to those of the third and last Order, to wit, by the Secret Menstruums of the Antients.

CHAP.

CHAP. V.

Of the Secret Menſtruums *of the Antients,* viz. *Their* Acetum, Spirit of *Wine*, Liquor Alkaheſt *and* Sal Panariſtos.

IN this Chapter, I ſhall for the benefit of thoſe deſirous of Learning give an *Eſſay* to all theſe, which being underſtood, will highly contribute to the diſcovery of all the Miſterious Medicines of the Antients, which hitherto have been folded up in Tropes, and Metaphors, Ænigmatical Speeches, and Parabolical Sayings; yet contained in one thing, or ſubject Matter, only diverſified by different Operations into different Effects, ſome more eaſie, ſome more hard to be obtained: But before I can diſtinctly particularize theſe, I think it convenient to deſcribe their Source or Fountain.

For the Foundation of theſe, as I told you *in my laſt Edition*, there is a *General Chaos*, which the Philoſophers have deſcribed, containing a Spermatick Eſſence of all Created Beings, as alſo the three firſt pure Principles of Minerals and Metals; ſo that this is a Book of wonder, the Looking-glaſs of Nature, wherein may be diſcerned ſo many Miſteries, that I have neither time, nor in this ſmall compaſs,

compaſs, room to ſet them forth; therefore I ſhall only ſpeak Practically of that Part, which will make what I have promiſed compleat and perfect; and this in ſuch words, as peradventure has not been written from the Foundation of the World; intending to do that here, which has been omitted by the Philoſophers in General.

Take the known Animal, Vegetable and Mineral Matter, called *Bitumen Mundi*, and having diſtill'd the Superior and Inferior Waters, bring to Calcination by its proper Fire; extract the Salt, as the true Foundation of Art; but this is not that Salt I call *Sal Panariſtos*, but that Ground, in which the Seed is to be putrified for the obtaining of it: Therefore having ſeparated the Superior and inferior Waters, and the latter from all Poiſonous, Arſenical, Coagulating Salts, is to be united to the foreſaid Salt, and dried by the regular Courſe of Nature, and then conjoined with the white and red, Male and Female Earth, Subliming the *Mercury* from the *Armoniack*; for *Artephius* tells you, 'tis ſo obtain'd; for this you have a Key that opens the Door of Entrance, both to Medicine and Alchimy: For if you unite the Superior Waters with its proper Earth, of which there be two ſorts, white, and red, concerning which St. *Duſtan* bids you *ſow a white in the white, and a red in the red*; the Water having taken on the Nature of that Sulphur, or Body, then aſſatiate with the Vinegar and Sublimate; and ſo by deco-

cting

ſting in this tripple Veſſel, you obtain both Body and Blood; the Body muſt remain it its Station, as the Foundation of the Work, and Veſſel of Nature; but the Blood is to be united with the Mercurial and Paſſive Elements of Earth and Water; for both their Concretion, Exaltation and Purification; for they are both Concoagulated, and become one Homogeneous *Menſtruum*, which is our *Vinegar* and *Philoſophical Spirit* of *Wine*, the one being aqueous and clear, the other of an oily and creamy Subſtance: But be ſure in the Sublimation that you force not the Fire too long; for when the white fume aſcends, change your Receiver, for 'tis the red devouring Dragon that muſt be ſeparated apart; but the Salt that follows is more precious: Here adding to the Doctrine of the Philoſophers, you have Mercury ſeparated from its watry Aquoſity and Terrene *Fæces*; but be not ſo ſtupid to think this the Mercury of Philoſophers, but the firſt Matter or Agent, by which they prepare their Mercury by ſeveral Animations; for the Matter goes through various States, as *Philalethes* ſays, before the Kingly Diadem is caſt out of the *Menſtruum* of the common Harlot, and ſo accordingly receives its Name, as *Chaos*, *Arſenick*, *Air*, *Lune*, *Magnet*, *Chalybs* or *Steel*, *Green-lyon*, and many others, too numerous to name. Therefore be ſure this white and living *Gur* is the Sperm of Metals which muſt be nouriſhed in the lap of Nature, even in the Philoſophers Heaven; where it will

will be imbraced, and by its Spiritual Seed this Virgin Nature will conceive and bring forth a Son, which is neither Corporal nor Spiritual, but of a middle Nature, between Heaven and Earth; ponderous in respect of Heaven, as an active form; but light in respect to Earth, as passive, yet carries the Golden Chain which unites Heaven and Earth together; and therefore returning him again upon the Earth, unite him with such things as will make him undergo all mortal Torments of Death and Mortification; that so by Regeneration he may be qualify'd to return to Heaven again: This circular Motion you continue 'till the Heaven has impregnated the Earth with its Validity, so as to bring forth the slimosity of Elements, or that Dust of which *Adam* was formed, which being endued with a Vegetative and living Soul, *Eve* the first Woman, is taken as a Rib from *Adam*; for the Body is divided into two parts, one to wash and cleanse, the other to be washed and cleansed; therefore by this Central Mercurial *Medium*, one half of the Body being distil'd, and its Spirits taken in the Heavenly Region, you shall obtain *Azoth* and *Laton*, or *Adam* and *Eve*, one in the upper part, the other in the lower, as Philosophers say; and tho' *Laton* is an impure Body, yet it is cleansed by *Azoth*, and separated from all its Aquosity and Earthy Combust *Faces*, his Eyes then shining like Lightning, and his Face like a flame of Fire; for the Spirit makes the Body like molten

ten Glaſs which no other thing but the Sword of the Spirit can do, as being the Son of Heaven, that preſerves the Tree of Life from all that which is not regenerated by the Water and Spirit of *Prima Materia*: But I ſhall paſs by this, leaving the *Sophi* to injoy their own Gifts, in that I neither intend to ſet up for a Philoſopher, nor to become a profeſs'd Adept, having already too much intruded upon the Learning of theſe good Men; for 'tis my buſineſs to advance the Medicinal Art, by letting the ſincere deſirer know that theſe Principles being united in their party, will Chryſtalize into a Salt, which is that wonderful Salt I call **Sal Panariſtos**, of whoſe Medicinal Vertues whole Volums might be written; yet nevertheleſs I am not ignorant that the Philoſophers Intention was to prepare one *Panacea*, by ſeparating their pure Principles into a Salt, Sulphur and Mercury, *viz.* A white Incombuſtible Oil, a red Incombuſtible Oil, and pure Diamond Powder Salt, of which this Medicine is afterward compounded; what is further to be ſaid of this here, and particularly of the *Fires* and *Menſtruums*, take as follows.

In

In Laudem Trium Sophicorum Ignium.

Heat, that produces all things, must prepare
Their Bodies, and disclose what Forms they
(wear,
By Fire, the Sovereign Element, we thence
A Vinegar derive, no Friend to Sence,
Nor flatt'rer of the Palate, 'tis compos'd
Of Earth and Water, amicably clos'd;
Thence it dissolves to Water, and the white
Sublimate Sal-Armoniack, *which unite*
Into Earths White and red, and Mercur,
To form the Prior Body does comply,
And Tripple Vessel of Philosophy:
The Blood, that fiery Dragon *qualifies,*
And makes to the Mercurial Vessel rise;
And thence the Female Dragon *does proceed,*
Who to the Male *must afterwards recede:*
As Nature in the Orb does circulate
By sending (order'd by the Laws of Fate)
The Spermy Doses *to the Earth, which sink,*
And thence the Sun does rising moisture drink;
And leaves the multiplying Sperm, which does
Proceed on Bodies; 'tis the way that's chose
By Nature, and her Circulation shows.
Three Eagles *do resemble it, and shew*
The Compound Vinegar's *free* Medium *true*
Is Complicate, and is the Medium *there,*
By which the Blood and Body strengthen'd are,
The one its Central Spirit does allow,
The other does its vital Life bestow;

And both combine together to produce
Our Second Fire of Philosophick use;
Thence the Third Fire, the Mountain's Floody (Sperm
Is freed; and this we Artfully affirm;
Unvail'd, unbound, from Earthly Chains set free,
This third most sacred Fire the Sophi see;
Which Azoth some, but others do it name
The Lyon Green, well known in Rolls of Fame;
By which they do their Sun and Moon conjoyn,
And Natures actions with Nature do Combine:
By this are clip'd the swift Cyllenian Wings;
The Body this to Dissolution brings;
By this moist Heat the Sun and Moon descend,
And all their Vertues downward it attend,
These downward drawn afford a lovely sight,
While in the Blood and Body they unite;
And under these two Forms when they come near,
Far stronger than before they then appear;
Since in the Triune Fountain we behold
What e'er in Mystick Fable we are told,
Of that fierce fiery Colchian Beast,
Within whose Bowels Treasures hid do rest;
Who doth the Magi's Chalybs there conceal,
Which worthy is of Wisdom to reveal:
Th' Elixir gives our Second Fire compleat,
The Volatile is fixed by its Heat;
Nor of Addition is here any need,
Besides it can produce a living Seed;
The living Seed of Metals here does lye,
Not dead, discover'd by the Artists Eye,
This is that Gur, that noble Lunar Oyl,
For which so many vainly rove and toyl;

Th.

This Fire it is which made **Pontanus** wise,
The Fire, which made Artephius *so to rise.*
In Years, and all the living Weights excel;
For nothing can its mighty force repel:
From Sulphur is its Birth; but make not hast,
If you wou'd not your Time and Labour wast;
Since from the Matter this you must not take,
For it's a Sulphur *of another make:*
But when the Blood and Mercury you have found,
And it by dextrous hidden Art have bound;
Then Nature learn sweetly to imitate,
As she will teach you how to circulate;
In her Circulations your Pattern see
Always; and from this Pattern never flee:
This now to animate and fortifie,
Eagles, be sure, you must seven more let fly;
By every flight the Light begets a day,
While Darkness from the Light makes hast away;
In every one a Separation's made,
The vanquish'd Darkness now can't make afraid;
For see, behold the Splendour that appears;
See the bright Nymph, that here her Head uprears;
A living Splendent Fountain now doth run,
With a Transcendent Brightness, as the Sun,
Shining and streaming Vertue all a-round,
By which it penetrates whole Nature's Ground;
This, as the Azoth *true, our living Spring,*
The Body to Perfection soon will bring:
Here Laton, *melted, open'd and calcin'd,*
By this Mercurial Fire is refin'd;
Laton, *our Gold, here many times baptize,*
We do imbibe and wash, till to its size
And Standard true, it do at last arrive,
For which it will be worth our while to strive;

Nor is there loss of any other part,
But all remains, not touch'd, nor chang'd by Art:
For this Immortal Fiery Liquor's such,
As nought can ever change, or ever touch;
This with the Matter cannot alter'd be;
By it the Matter alter'd we shall see;
So as thereby to be transparent quite,
And thus made almost of a radiant white;
Which to the Nature of a Spirit turns,
While it in Spirit unconsumed burns:
The Spirit with the Body thus conjoyn'd,
We thence a most excelling Creature find;
In which a Trine of Principles doth lye,
Pure Salt, pure Sulphur and pure Mercury;
These Art can separate, and then unite;
That Art of which the hidden Sophi write,
But none besides, none but Dame Nature's Art,
This wondrous Secret ever did impart:
Within this Mine two Stones of old were found,
Whence this the Antients called Holy Ground;
Who knew their Value, Power and Extent,
And Nature how with Nature to Ferment
For these if you Ferment with Nat'ral Gold
Or Silver, their hid Treasures they unfold,
According to their Natures then proceed,
And take care properly each one to feed;
Imbibe, Multiply, and when you project,
Then shall be seen the wonderful Effect;
Which may indeed the ignorant amaze,
Not so the Wise, who will not vainly gaze;
But falling prostrate down will God adore
And joyful offer up to him their Store.

Amen.

Thus

Thus, Reader, I have in general describ'd our *Menstruums* and *Fires*, which being rightly understood, may serve as a Guide to the *Mount Helicon* of *Art*, especially to such as will make Coales, Glasses and hard Labour their Interpreters; yet for the benefit of such, I shall be a little more particular, in giving some general Hints concerning the Matter and Preparation of the great *Hilech*, or the *Circulatum Minus* of *Paracelsus*, called by his great Interpreter *Van Helmont*, *Alkahest*, from the *German* word *Al-gehest*, which signifies *All Spirit*; because after its Preparation no corporal Matter remains in it; the Preparation of this being abundantly more difficult than any other Chymical *Arcanum*; for as *Philalethes* says, *'tis an hundred times more difficult to prepare than the Grand Elixir*; and a principal Reason is, because the true Matter and manner of its Preparation is not conceived from the Writings of the Antients; and so every conceited Ideot, who is fill'd with the airy Notions of a phantistick Brain, grounds his own Opinion for Truth, and slights all others as fallacious; being too full to be taught; of this number are the *Mercury* and *Regulus-mongers*, and the Doters on Vitriol, Salts and imperfect Metals, which I can no better compare than to the *Saxon Chymist* in his new Spagyrical Chymistry, who in one Paragraph affirms and denies, and yet condemns the Authority of the Antients, because he does not understand them; and yet at the ſame time would allude, that he himſelf were Maſter of ſome great Myſteries: What I have to ſay of this Point, is, that ſuch a *Chaos* and Hodg-podg is fit for ſuch Operators; and long may they hug and injoy them, as not being qualified for receiving Truth in its Innocency; therefore I think I ſhould do them much wrong, if I ſhould ſeek to convince them of their Errors; for I never ſtrove to do it, when I have met with abundance of thoſe *German* Chymiſts in my Travels; their Heads being like their Clock-work, abundance of Motions, too much incumber'd to perform true Time, and too chargable to be kept; ſo that they are become as uſeleſs in moſt parts of *Europe*, as their airy Chymiſts. But to return from this Digreſſion to the Matter in hand; which is to lay down the Fundamental Grounds of the beſt Authors, who have treated of the *Liquor Alkaheſt*, beginning firſt with *Paracelſus*; tho' I cannot conceive that he has deſcribed the Matter any more than by the Scope of its Tendency; for it muſt be Univerſal, ſeeing he declares the Vertue and Office of his *Liquor* to be ſo, when prepared; neither indeed has he been any clearer in his Preparation, ſeeing what he has given concerning it, is only that of Solution and Coagulation, where he bids you diſſolve from its Coagulated State, and Coagulate again into a tranſmuted Form.

Now this of Solution and Coagulation, being a Proceſs alike, and common to moſt

Chy-

Chymical Processes, there is so little Information to be gathered from what he has said, that we shall here pass it by, and come to his great Expositor *Van Helmont.*

Helmont, when he comes to describe this *Liquor*, tells us, 'tis found in a *Latex*, which is an hidden Source or Fountain, and is a Body of Salt, appearing under two *Faces* or Forms, which he says must be reduced to one, to make Symphony or Harmony; which words are obscure enough, and the Process he gives as equally dark, being only that of reiterated Solution and Intervening Coagulation, and so to reduce it into the smallest Attoms possible in Nature; which he describes by the Serpent biting himself, reviving from that Poison, and thenceforth becomes Immortal.

Starkey seems to agree with this Process of *Helmont*, and to Illustrate it; but he, *in his Treatise of the Liquor Alkahest*, lays down human Urine, as its *Basis*, quoting his Authority from *Helmont*, where he gives this Encomy on this Salt, *viz.* That it excels all other particular Salts there reckon'd up; and when he comes to give the Process of the *Alkahest*, says, *'tis the subtil penetrating Spirit of Human Urine, united with that which is centrally one with it*; which he proves to be a Vinous Spirit and Oil; saying, 'tis done by means of an Acid, not Corrosive, but grateful to Nature; and by often Circulation attains to that height of Purity, as to be call'd *Ens Salium*, *Summum Salium Principium*: As the Matter here

R 4 de-

deſcribed is in Terms alien and obſcure, ſo is his Proceſs but little clearer ; for in another place he ſays, 'tis made by long digeſtion, it being ſome days before bereaved of its Coagulating Spirit ; and in the foreſaid Proceſs he ſays, it obtains the height of its Purity by often Circulation, which if he underſtood what he ſaid, theſe Expreſſions are far more wide and obſcure than the other.

But *Philalethes* in his Treatiſe extant, grounds his Proceſs on Blood and Urine, and bids you take Urine, and putrifie it, not in a Glaſs, but earthen Veſſel, ſix Weeks, light cloſed or cover'd ; and by the Addition of *Salt Nitre*, draw from it a Spirit ſomewhat Vinous, which he ſays is wonderful in the Diſſolution of Bodies, but cannot ſubſiſt without Blood ; aſſerting that in Urine, and Blood the *Alkahest* lies hid : To compleat his Proceſs, he bids you to take the Salt of new Urine, and gently evaporate to a drineſs, diſſolve in half ſo much Water, Filtrate, congeal and diſſolve, and then Cohobate till all is come over.

This Proceſs, tho' it carries Clearneſs and Truth in it to a Son of Art, yet it is abſtruſe and obſcure enough to thoſe who underſtand not his Analogy, becauſe by the Urine and Blood, here expreſſed, he means that of the great World, the Matter being originally the ſame with that of the great *Elixir*, as may be eaſily conceived from his other Writings For where he ſpeaks of the force of the *Fiery Dragon*, or *Blood*, he ſays, it overcomes all things, that is to ſay, when diſtill'd ſtill'd with the Mercurial Salt; but in the way of Generation the Vegetable *Saturnia* overcomes it; and 'tis clear from his Words in his *Introit. Apert.* p. 25. Where he treats of the Invention of the perfect Magiſtery, that theſe two have one Root; for *they rejected all Salts* (ſays he) *one Salt only excepted, which is the firſt* Ens *of Salts, the which diſſolves all Metals, and by the ſame Work coagulates common Mercury; but it is done, but in a violent way, and therefore that kind of Agent is again ſeparated entire, both in Weight and Vertue from the things it is put to.*

And *in his Expoſition on Sir* George Ripley'*s Epiſtle*, he ſhews, that Alkalies make a violent Separation between the Sulphur and Mercury; but here you may conceive that he points forth our Univerſal Alkaly, which is an Agent in preparing the *Immortal Liquor*; which you may in part gather from what is ſaid, does proceed from the ſame Root as the grand *Elixir*; but for a full Confirmation, hear what *Ludovicus de Comit.* ſays.

Ludovicus de Comit: That thrice Noble and unparallel'd Son of Art was the very firſt that gave me the Satisfaction in this Point; not only ſo, but a large inſight into the Operation it ſelf, where he ſays, *The Foundation Matter of the Grand Elixer and Liquor Alkaheſt are all one, but diverſified by different Operations to different Effects; one being purely Natural. the other Artificial*; he gives you an Example of this by a Grain of Corn, of its being ſown in its

its own Matrix, to wit, the Earth, or fermented and brought into Spirit, in which the Seminal Vertue is totally Annihilated: Now the Sowing of *Sol* in its own Mercurial Matrix is Generative and Natural; but fermenting the Body with ☉, ⊕ and * and violently distilling into a Spirit, is forcible, which being effected, the Gold can never be reduced to a Body: Therefore, *Philalethes* says, there is no Congelation by evaporating its moisture, the Liquor being Spiritual and Uniform, being neither Acid nor Alcaly, but an unctious oily Salt, that gives its flegm out first, but to bring it to this state is exceeding difficult; for as *Philalethes* himself confesses, its Preparation is an hundred times more difficult than that of the great *Elixir*, yet is not so candid to tell us what these difficulties are; but my Friend *Ludovicus* has clearly hinted them under these three Heads: The first, is, as the Preparation of this Liquor is purely Artificial, so is it variously to be conceived of, seeing the true Process is but one; to wit, Solution and intervening Coagulation: The second, is, as its Preparation is forcible and violent (for the Principles are distill'd into Spirits, and so being separated from the strict tye they had in the Elements, they become weaker a second time, and rather pass away into fume, than come again to Coagulation (as I know experimentally) if you know not how to coagulate and keep it in by a friendly help) so to effect this point is the most diffi-

difficult thing in the World. The third difficulty, is, the Separation of things adjoyned, which are a Sulphureous Combuſt Oil, Terrene *Faces* and an Aqueous Flegm ; for as in the violent diſſolution it is reduc'd to the ſmalleſt parts, ſo is it endowed with an active diſſolving Quality, reducing things to their firſt matter, which is Aqueous ; ſo in the Preparation great quantities of Flegm ſeparate from it, which the Liquor will rather paſs over with, than come again to a true Coagulation ; nay, ſome of the Flegms are ſo inherent, if Salts are added to break the Body, that they will bear the ſame degree of Fire as the *Alkaheſt*, and come over with it, which you muſt carefully ſeparate in every Operation ; for theſe Flegms are its Compeer, or water, by which it is deſtroy'd ; for being joyned with it, you ſhall never ſee its fiery diſſolving Vertue ; therefore, Art and Patience muſt be made uſe of, to bring it to a State of Retrogradation, or a going back to Coagulation ; which, as *Ludovicus* ſays, is impoſſible to be done without the concurring help of an Aſſiſtant.

From what has been ſaid, it may be eaſily conceived, that the Univerſal Matter, whence *Paracelſus* prepared his *Alkaheſt*, was the Philoſophers *Chaos*, which is one with *Helmont's Latex*, and the two Faces which this Liquor in the firſt manifeſtation appears under, is the Body and Blood ; which ſome for the likeneſs in Operation, call Urine and Spirit of Wine ;

Wine; *Philalethes*, Urine and Blood; but we with *Ludovicus* call them the Central Waters and Blood, or Spirit of the Blood; one being brought to a Vinous and Mineral Spirit, the other to a Urinous; which being united, do not only bring about Immortality, but also enable the Artist reasonably to reconcile all those different Allegorical Expressions which Authors have delivered concerning it.

This at present may suffice concerning the Theory, having written a particular Treatise of this Immortal Liquor, wherein these things are more amply shewn; but the Bookseller having contrary to his Agreement kept it from the light, I think it not amiss to give a short Recapitulation of the Practice, and so conclude.

In the first place, you may observe, that the Matter is one with the Universal Medicine, but by different Operations brought to different effects: *Secondly*, the Preparation of the *Mercury* of *Philosophers*, is purely Natural; but of this *Immortal Dissolvent*, wholly Artificial, and therefore exceeding difficult, and the more in that you have to do with a Subject, which *Proteus-like*, takes on all forms, and so rather passes over, than comes again to Coagulation. *Thirdly*, it is prepared by the *Dragon* devouring his own Tail, and then renewing into that State, over which Death has no Power, his Transmutation being then as impossible as washing the Blackamore white; because

cause the Body of Salts of two Faces is brought to Purity and Consenting Harmony, which for the future is liable to no Corruption nor Dissipation of Parts: *Lastly*, to sum up all, I say 'tis impossible to obtain this *Liquor*, but by diligent search and hard Labour, because the Process of its Preparation was never given by the Antients; therefore you must trace the way step by step, with convenient Glasses and Furnaces, and be armed with Patience for all Disappointments; otherwise 'tis never to be obtained by the most piercing Wit in the World; for as *Helmont* says, *God sells Art for Labour*, and cries out, *God knows the reason, why he has given the Goat so short a Tail*; and further, *O! that I had removed my Receiver*; by which I find he came to loss, as I my self have sometimes done.

Thus I have been more large in the Description of this *Immortal Liquor*, its Utility being so great, when prepared; for by it the chief Medicinal Mysteries are obtained, the true knowledge of which, from the Minority of my Study I ever more desired, than that of transmuting the imperfect into perfect Metals; and therefore have I taken all these pains for the Caution and Instruction of the Industrious, having compiled, *Tyro-like*, that in a small compass, which the Crafty Masters have strewed in their large Volums: Therefore my sincere desire is, that the industrious Reader may receive the Benefit designed by the Author, so concluding these, shall come in the next to shew its use.

CHAP.

CHAP. VI.

Officium Generale Circulati Minoris in Preparatione Magisteriorum, Essentiarum & Quintessentiarum.

The Office of the Circulatum Minus, in Preparing Magisteries, Essences and Quintessences in General.

NOW as we have before denied any of these to be prepared without the help of the *Universal Medium*, which being in it self exalted, so as to become an active *Menstruum*, we shall now come to show the Practical Office thereof in the Preparing of the afore-named and first of the Magisteries.

A **Magistery** signifies a principal Master-piece in Art, and is the *Calx* of any Metal so dissolved by the Fire of Nature, as that it becomes fusible like Wax, and will admit of its Sulphur and Mercury to be separated, in order that they may be brought to their primitive Juice and pure State, or the Universal Principles so reduced. *Example*, Take the Calx of any of the imperfect Metals, whether *Saturn*, *Jupiter*, &c. Or of the Minerals, as *Antimony*, *Spelter* or the *Metallum Magnum Paracelsi*, or of the more perfect Metals,

Metals, as *Mars*, *Venus*, *Lune*, or *Sol*, and put the *Circulatum Minus* on it in treble weight; and this Fire being distill'd from any Metal, soft and imperfect, doth at the first or second time leave it in a fusible Substance, like Wax: But for the harder Metals, you must repeat it three, four, or five times; then have you the Metal or Mineral left like a sweet Salt, of a fragrant Scent, potable in any Liquor, and will yield its Tincture, if dissolved in pure Spirit of Wine; whence you may easily obtain the Magistery: But if you will proceed further, the Tincture being taken, the residue must be kept three days in a vaporous Heat, and a quick and running Mercury may be separated; and the Saline Power being truly obtained, may be united with the aforesaid Tincture: These Magisteries are indued with Vertues, according to their Specifick Power: *That of Saturn is an Anodyne, cooling Inflamations, resolving Tumors, and stopping Gonorrhaas, the Dose from three to eight, and sometimes sixteen or twenty drops: That of Jupiter is excellent in Suffocations of the Womb, old Sores, Cancers and Fistulaes; the Dose is the same with the former: That of the Mettallum Masculum, or Spelter cures the most Herculean Diseases that contemn to stoop to other Medicines; the Dose is from six to twelve, sometimes eighteen drops. The Magistery of Lune and Sol is prepared the same way, its Vertue may be conceived from that of Poable Sol and Lune.*

An

An **Essence** is the Substance of any Body dissolved by this Liquor, and often cohobated till the whole is exalted to a Spiritual State, that is the purer Sulphur, separated and brought into a Spiritual Essence, the which you may do not only by any of the aforesaid Metals, but even by the Universal it self.

A **Quintessence** is the Metallick *Calx*, so long Cohobated until it is brought over, as you may see in the *Aurum Potabile*; as also the Elements or Principles destroyed of their Qualities, and a fifth Power Extracted, which is wholly Glorious, Vital and Spiritual; so is Heaven the Quintessence of all the Elements, yea, even of the whole Creation, thence so far excels in Beauty.

Elixir (as aforesaid) signifies such an Universal Medium, as will by its Cælestial Purity and Tinging Sulphur change and transmute imperfect Beings in the smallest parts into a State of Perfection.

Panacæa signifies a Medicine which hath Power in it self to cure all Diseases; therefore what this said Menstruum cannot upon Specificated Bodies perform, must be done by and through an higher Exaltation of the most Universal Principles, which indeed is the *Magistery* of *Hermes*; and therefore is *Magistery* a proper Name also for the *Grand Essence*, as well as for such Metallick Bodies as are dissolved by the Circulatum Minus, so that all these proceed from this *Medium's* help, or from a true Exaltation of the first Principles in in themſelves; for this Reaſon we eſteem it a Foppery in thoſe that call thoſe things Magiſteries that have not the leaſt adherence thereunto, as the *Magiſtery* of *Pearl*, *Oyſter-ſhells*, &c. When alas they are all the while ignorant of the *Menſtruum*, by which the whole Body of the *Calx* is diſſolved, ſo as to be brought into a ſweet Salt, giving up its Vertue in any Liquor (as aforeſaid) and are like to remain ſo until they learn a better Leſſon of Dame Nature, who muſt acquaint them with the aforeſaid Menſtruum, which will be inſtrumental to unlock many *Arcanums* for the true Spagyriſt, not ſuch as the Pſeudo-Chymiſts of this Age eſteem for ſuch, but thoſe which have their Preparation through, or Foundation from the Univerſal Powers of Nature, and ſuch as have neither of theſe cannot be eſteemed ſo, whatever the great Impoſtours may be pleaſed to ſtile their Slop-Preparations, in order to deceive the half blinded World; nay, without this Menſtruum the Eſſential and Genuine Powers of Bodies are not to be prepared; for 'tis thro' radical Diſſolution that things are brought to a pure State, for being Spiritualized, what they are virtuouſly impowered withal will be manifeſtly ſhown in the Act, and ſome in a way ſuperior to others: And there are Medicines in Nature of ſuch univerſal Tendency, as that they cure Diſeaſes without having regard to Age, Sex or Conſtitution; nay, further than this, make Renovation even to youthful

S Strength

Strength and Vigour; of which Nature is the Grand *Aurum Potabile* of the Adepts: But this being touch'd at elsewhere, we shall here omit it, and come to the more particular use of this Menstruum.

Lilium Antimonii Nostrum, *or, our Lily of Antimony.*

℞ Antimonial Flowers sublimed through *Sal-Armoniack*, the Salt being edulcorated, or wash'd therefrom; or the Alcool of Antimony brought to a *Calx* or *Scory*, and the Salts by which 'tis performed, being again washed therefrom, and then on a Marble Ground to an impalpable Powder; of either of these take ℥ii, of the *Circulatum Minus* ℥iv, digest 6 or 8 hours, and then distil off the Dissolvent, and you shall have a true *Precipiolum*, the which edulcorate, and so is it prepared.

Its Vertues.

'Tis a prevalent **Arcanum** *in Dropsies, and Purges the Blood of all Watry Humours: The Dose is from 6 to 12 Grains, with the fine Powder, or rather the Rosin of Jallop.*

Magi-

Magisterium Saturni, *or, the Magistery of Saturn.*

℞. Of the *Calx* of *Saturn* one part, of the *Circulatum Minus* two parts, digest twenty four hours, and then draw off your Dissolvent, and extract the Tincture (which will be blood-red and sweet) with Spirit of Wine, which is the Magistery.

Its Vertues.

'Tis (as we said before) an Anodyne, Cooling Inflamations, Resolving Tumors, Curing Gangrenes, and stopping Gonorrhœas: The Dose is from 3 to 8, sometimes 16 or 20 drops in a Glass of Wine.

Thus may be made the Magistery of *Jupiter* and *Mars*, &c.

Magisterium Solare & Aurum Potabile, *or, the Magistery of Gold, Potable in any Liquor.*

We have given you one in *Page* 133, of our *Chymicus Rationalis*, which is the Gold Calcin'd by our *Sal Panaristos*, and the Vertue extracted by the Volatile and Genuine Spirit of Tartar, and lastly in Spirit of Wine, which is a Noble Preparation; but however we ſhall add others that are wholly prepared by the *Circulatum Minus.*

℞. Fine Gold and Calcine it into ſmall Attoms, or laminate it into thin Leaves, then put it into a ſmall Retort, and pour upon it three times its weight of the aforeſaid *Menſtruum,* and in a boiling heat, being exactly ſtopt, let it remain fourteen or fifteen days, and it will be diſſolved in the Liquor without any ſediment; then the Liquor being diſtil'd off, 'twill be left in form of a fuſible Salt, as we ſaid in other Magiſteries, which is a Medicine *moſt eminent againſt the Palſie, and all Malignant Feavers, the Plague and Peſtilence*: But if you'll proceed to its higheſt Exaltation, it muſt be brought over the Helm, which is performed by often, at leaſt ten or fifteen Cohobations with the ſame Liquor, until the whole Body of the Gold is made Volatile, and comes over in two Colours, White and Red, and the Red is the *Hematine Tincture,* and the White may be reduced into a White Mercurial Body, after the diſſolving Liquor is ſeparated from the ſame: This is the higheſt Preparation of Gold that can be made by this Liquor, it being its Eſſence, *and hath Power to Cure the moſt Refractory and Deplorable Diſeaſes incident to Human-kind: Its Doſe is from one drop to five or ſix at the moſt in a Glaſs of Wine.*

Or

Or thus, ℞. Of the *Calx* of Gold ℥i, and of the *Circulatum Minus* ℥iii, put them into a long neck'd Viol, and digest for the space of three days, or until it will give no more Tincture, which being done, pour out the Solution into a Retort, and with a gentle Fire Distil off the Dissolving Liquor, and from the Golden Solution remaining in the Retort, Extract an aurified Tincture with Spirit of Wine, and so have you a true *Aurum Potabile*: The same Process may be observed in *Venus*, *Silver*, or others. Observe, that *Lune* thus made Potable is *a Specifick in the Falling-sickness, strengthning the Head and Animal Spirits: The Dose is from 5 to 12 drops.*

Magisterium Mercury & Arcanum Corallinum, *or, the Magistery of Mercury and Coralline Secret.*

℞. Of the true Precipitate of Mercury, well edulcorated, made after what manner you will, ℥i, and of the *Circulatum Minus* ℥iii, digest twenty four hours, then distil off the Dissolvent, and you will have a fixed Precipitate, upon which the *Menstruum* being Cohobated two or three times, 'twill be made more fusible, and the easier admit of its pure Principles to be taken in Spirit of Wine, which is the true Magistery: Or if this fix'd Precipitate is wash'd with Water of the Whites of Eggs 'twill become red, or thus,

Diaceltateſſon Noſtrum, *or, our Diaceltateſſon.*

℞. Of Mercury vulgar one part, of the aforeſaid *Menſtruum* two parts; diſtil of your *Menſtruum*, and repeat this a ſecond time, and ſo will you find the Body left coagulated and fixed, ſo as to indure the Teſt of *Saturn*; 'tis left Spongious like to a Pumice-ſtone, but heavy like *Turbith Mineral*, brittle, and therefore without difficulty Pulverizable, which then being cohobated with Water diſtill'd from whites of Eggs, cauſeth that diſtill'd Water to ſtink, but becomes of the colour of the beſt Coral; that which *Helmont* prepared by his *Alkaheſt*, was called by him *Arcanum Corallinum* ſo indeed may either of theſe; however here we with *Paracelſus* and *Starkey*, *Diaceltateſſon.*

Its Vertues.

Either of theſe is a certain, ſure and ſafe Arcanum to relieve in Plagues, Feavers, Dropſie, Scurvey, Gout and Stone, The Doſe is from three to five, ſometimes ſeven or nine Grains.

Thus having run through the Metals, we ſhall now come to the Minerals, and firſt of Vitriol.

Oleum

Oleum Anodynum Veneris, *or, the Anodyne Oyle of* Venus.

℞. Of the Vitriol of *Venus*, or the best Roman Vitriol, Calcine it till it be throughly wasted what will wast, then dulcifie the Colcothar with pure Water, and dry it; to this being dried, put double the quantity of our *Circulatum Minus*, and 'twill easily and speedily be dissolved, distil off your *Menstruum*, and return it back again, and Cohobate it at the least twelve or fourteen times so will all the Body of the Colchothar be brought over the Helm in form of a green Liquor; digest this in a gentle Heat of *Balneum* for about a Month, and then distil it in a slow Fire, so will the whole Metalline Substance of the *Venus* come over, leaving the *Menstruum* below in the bottom of the Retort in its intire *Pondus* and Vertue: To this Liquor or Spirit come over, put an equal quantity of *Sal-Armoniack*, dissolved in as much Water as will dissolve it, so shall you separate the green Liquor from a white Sediment, which white Sediment will give a white Metal, as fix'd as Silver, and which will abide the Test of *Saturn*, but yet formally distinct from Silver, which thou (if a Philosopher) shall easily perceive, however as good to a Metallurgist as the best Silver; the green Liquor dry up in a Viol Glass, by evaporating all the moisture, for it is the

Sulphur of the *Venus*, mixed with the *Sal-Armoniack*, by which, (note that) it is fixed, so that it will abide all Fire; this Sulphur extract with the pure Spirit of Wine which will dissolve it, leaving the *Sal Armoniack*; then distil away from it (thus dissolved) your Spirit of Wine, and you'll have left a very fragrant green Oil of *Venus*, which is the Sulphur of *Venus* Essentificated by these Operations, as sweet to tast as the best Honey, *than which Nature hath not a more Soveraign Remedy for most, (not to say all) Diseases: This is the* Nepenthe Verum *of the Philosophers before-mentioned, which causeth certain rest, and asswages all Pain, but ever after Sleep leaves the Party, either sensibly amended (in more violent and Diuternal Diseases) or quite well in the less rigid Maladies.*

The like doth the *Anodyne Oil of Mercury*, which is this *Menstruum* so long cohobated upon the fixed Precipitate until the whole Body is brought over, and the Sulphur is separated from the Central Mercury, and being truly exalted, *is in all violent Corruptions of the Blood, a more Soveraign Specifick and Arcanum than the former: The Dose of either of these is from 5 to twenty drops in a Glass of fragrant Wine.*

Aurum

Aurum Horizontale Nostrum, *or, our Horizontal Gold.*

The Preparation of an *Horizontal Gold* hath been touch'd at by *Van Helmont* and *Starkey*; the first intimates it to be the Sulphur of *Venus*, carried up by *Sal-Amoniacus Spagyricus*, and the *Sal-Armoniack* separated therefrom, and the *Sulphur* Dulcified, and then Cohobated upon Precipitate Vigo, until the Sulphur is fixed thereon; and this he calls *Aurum Horizontale*, or Gold in the Horizon; because it is fixed as Gold in the Fire: But the latter expresses this to be a Sulphur of *Venus*, prepared by the *Liquor Alkahest*, and separated from the white Metal, then Cohobated upon the aforesaid Precipitate 'till fixed: But we prepare it from the Sulphur of *Venus*, made by our aforesaid *Circulatum Minus*: But, now whether our said *Menstruum* is in all things the same with *Helmont*'s *Alkahest*. I shall not here assert, neither so much as dispute it; so that every one may remain in their Opinion, as we desire to do in the Preparation and Use of this *Menstruum*, which will in the Medicinal part perform all that we desire therefrom; now to the exact *Modus* in preparing the *Horizontal Gold*.

℞. Of the *Precipitate Vigo*, or any of the afore-named Percipitates one part; of this Sulphur of *Venus* two parts, put it into a

Re-

Retort and draw off the Sulphur what will come over, Cohobate it back again, and repeat this Operation so long as 'twill imbrace any Sulphur; and at last give it a strong degree of Fire, by which means it becomes as fixed as Gold and pleasant, from which (if you please) you may burn Spirit of Wine two or three times, so it is prepared.

Its Vertues.

This being taken inwardly, doth with few Doses cure the most desperate Diseases, either inward or outward, to which mans Nature is subject; as the Leprosie, Gout, Palsie, Epilepsie, Cancers, Fistulaes, Wolves, Scurvy, King's-evil, Venereal Disease &c. *And with one Dose cures all Feavers and Agues, the Hectick only excepted, which it cures in a Month; as also any sort of Consumption, and (in a word) is a perfect Remedy for any Malady prevailing over all, but Death, which (yet by curing all the Miseries of Life which reach the Health) it makes less truculent and dreadful.*

This Liquor also brings all Stones, Calxes and Shells, so as that they are potable in any Liquor, whence you may easily obtain their Magisteries, as for Example.

Magi-

Magiſterium Lithontripticum Maximum, *or, the whole Body of the* **Ludus** *brought into an Oil per deliq.*

℞. The Stone Ludus (what it is, and where to be found, *Helmont* exactly deſcribes) or in defect of that, take a Sand colour'd Flint, pulverize it exceeding fine, and pour thereon double its weight of our *Circulatum Minus*, draw it off, and the Stone will be diſſolved into a fuſible Subſtance, which being put into a moiſt place, let run *per deliquium*, and ſo it is prepared.

Its Vertues.

Of its Vertues none that have read **Helmont** *can be ignorant it radically cures the Gravel and Stone in the Kidneys and Bladder, and takes away all future Inclinations thereunto; The Doſe is twenty drops.*

Magiſterium Margaritæ, *or, the Magiſterial Milk, or Element of Pearl.*

℞. Pearl prepared ℥iii, of our *Circulatum Minus* ℥ix (or if ſcarce, ℥vi) digeſt and it will

will be diſſolved and brought into a Mucilage, reſolvable in Spirit of Wine: You may bring it into a Milk *per ſe*, which is its firſt *Ens*, or the Element of Pearl; after the ſame Way and Method may be made the *Magiſtery of Crab's-eyes*, but ſooner: Obſerve, *Starkey* ſays that theſe are not *Crab's-eyes*, but vulgarly ſo called, as being Stones found in the Head of the Crab.

Its Vertues.

'Tis excellent in the Anxieties of the Spleen and Scorbutick Cauſes, being alſo ſuperior in Vertue to the Milk of Crab's-eyes, eſpecially in Womens Diſeaſes: The Doſe is from eight to ſixteen drops.

Magiſterium Succini, *or, the Magiſtery of Amber.*

℞. Of the fineſt Amber one part, of our *Circulatum Minus* two parts, digeſt and draw off the Liquor, and the whole Body of the Amber will be diſſolved into a Saline and Fuſible Nature, which being taken in Spirit of Wine is the Magiſtery.

Its Vertues.

'Tis of admirable Vertue in Hypocondriack Melancholly and Uterine Diseases, and for Fits of all kinds: The Dose is from ten to thirty drops.

Elixir Proprietatis Paracelsi Alagistrale, *or, the Magisterial Elixir Proprietatis of Paracelsus.*

℞. Of Myrrh, Aloes and Saffron, ana. ℥i, of our aforesaid *Menstruum* ℥iii, digest in a gentle Heat and the whole will be dissolved, draw off your clear Liquor, and with pure Spirit of Wine extract the Magistery, which will be the whole Body of the *Species* into a Trifle: Now, if you design to make a quicker Dissolution, then let your Heat be stronger, and after the distilling off of your Liquor with the dissolved Body in a due Fire, so will the Oleous Sulphurous Part be turn'd into a Saline Spirit, which in a Distillation by Bath will come over in various colours, the *Crasis* separating it self from the Flegm (both by Colour, Tast and Smell, as also by its time of coming over the Helm distinguishable) and your Liquor left behind at bottom, as much in quantity, and as effectual in Vertue as before: But if you dissolve them in a Heat like to that of the Sun in the Spring, they being di-

diſtilled over and the Liquor ſeparated the Principles will ſeparate into an Aqueous Saline Liquor, and a more Sulphurous one. which digeſt in the like gentle heat, until the Oil and Water be united into an Eſſential Salt, which indeed is their firſt *Ens*: This mild way is that by which I adviſe you to prepare all Vegetables, eſpecially if you deſign to have their eminent Vertue, without looſing thoſe particular Excellencies which depend on the *Vita ultima* of the Concrete, otherwiſe a ſpeedier Preparation makes the Medicine no leſs effectual for curing Diſeaſes, though leſs powerful as to long Life.

Its Vertues.

'Tis a prevalent Medicine in Conſumptions, or any Waſting and Declining of the Body, for Phthiſick and ſhortneſs of Breath, and the like: 'Tis an excellent Antihectical Medicine, as alſo againſt Lypothymy's, Deliquia's, Convulſions, Palſies, &c *'Tis eſteemed moſt powerful for the prolonging of Life; but the firſt Ens of Cedar (according to* Helmont) is ſuperior to it; however this may take the next place, although the *Ens* of *Meliſſa* or *Bawme*, ſo prepared is not to be contemned: *The Doſe of this Magiſterial Ens in a Liquid Form is from* 3 *drops to nine, but in a Saline Form one Grain to five.*

Ob-

Obſerve, that after the ſame way may be made out of *Hellebore, a Noble Specifick againſt the Gout, Hypocondriack Melancholly, Calentures and Deliria's in Feavers*: And out of *Coloquintida an excellent Febrifuge; and out of Cortex Jeſuiticus an excellent Specifick againſt Agues of all kind, Quotidian, Tertian and Quartan*; and the like of other Concrets according to their Specifick Vertue: For you may clearly ſee that this Liquor diſſolves all Metals and Mineral Bodies, Gems, Pearls, Animals, Vegetables and Stones, Gums, Seeds and Roots; ſo that little more need be ſaid, ſeeing that by theſe Examples you may underſtand the reſt; and 'tis obſervable, in reſolving the Vegetables into their firſt Liquid Matter, that it diſtinguiſhes in them all their Heterogenieties by ſeveral Colours and diſtinct Places, one above another; in which Reſolution there always ſeats it ſelf in a diſtinct place a ſmall Liquor, eminently diſtinguiſhable from the reſt in Colour, in which the *Craſis* of the whole Herb, Tree or Seed doth reſide: For this agrees with what *Starkey* attributes to his *Liquor Alkaheſt*; and therefore as he ſaith, when any Concrete is made Retrograde by way of Diſſolution there is no loſs of Vertue, but an exalting of the ſame by many degrees, only whatever Virulency is in the Crude Concrete by this Operation is wholly extinct, with a Preſervation, notwithſtanding of all Specifick Vertues apparent

parent in the Concrete in its ſimplicity. Thus having repreſented unto you the uſe of this Liquor, as far as is needful, we ſhall here conclude with a few Examples, which may facilitate what is further deſired.

The Flowers of Sulphur being in this Liquor digeſted for the ſpace of two days, and then twice or thrice filtrated, they will paſs into the Form of a red Oil, ſeparate from the Liquor: which being ſeparated may be eſteemed as an Element of Fire of Sulphur, and is an excellent *Arcanum* for exalting Wines.

So likewiſe Cedar Wood being digeſted in a like proportion of the ſaid Liquor for the ſpace of twenty four Hours, the ſame will be wholly diſſolved, ſo that you may freely take its Vertue in Spirit of Wine; but if you proceed to exalt it to its firſt *Ens*, as we have directed in the *Elixir Proprietatis, then hath it the Vertues of promoting long Life*, as aforeſaid.

This Work alſo happily ſucceeds with Bawm, or any other Vegetable, (as aforeſaid, which is better to be uſed dry than freſh) being for ſome hours gently macerated in the Liquor.

Alſo

Alſo Charcoles are by it macerated and diſſolved, and (according to *Helmont*) the Work ſucceeds in all things for the bringing of it into its firſt Matter; but the Operation is changed and varied after a wonderful manner, according to the degree of the Fire and daily Digeſtion.

Nay, even Spirit of Wine being exactly Deflegmed and brought to the higheſt Subtilty, will by being digeſted in this Liquor be made yet more ſubtil and active, and more Homogeneous to Man's Body; nay, we ſuppoſe that this is that Spirit of Wine, mentioned by *Helmont*, which in two Hours will be converted into Arterial Blood, *&c.*

Thus having run through the Office of this Liquor in preparing of *Magiſteries*, *Eſſences*, *Quinteſſences*, and the moſt ſecret *Arcanums* of the moſt able Spagyriſts, we ſhall here conclude, and only add what is convenient for the Exaltation of Liquors and Artificial Brandies, which is principally from *Tartar*, *Sulphur* and *Venus*: For if the *Colcothar* of *Venus* is Volatilized by this our ſaid *Menſtruum*, then diſtill'd and brought over the Helm; the Sulphur being ſeparated from the Mercury, is then called the *Element* of *Fire* of *Venus*, and is an excellent *Arcanum* for meliorating Wines and

T Vinous

Vinous Spirits, being therein diluted; you must also know the Office of our *Sal Panaristos*, and by it to reduce common yellow Sulphur into a red fiery Stone which then will meliorate Wines, like that of the Sulphur of *Venus*; and if you put a little thereof into a Cask of Wine, the Wine acquires a grateful Tast and Odour, and will be so consolidated, as not easily to admit of changing or perishing, which otherwise so often happens to Wines, especially such as have not had their exalted maturity by the benevolent Raies of *Sol*, this Solar or Lunar Salt doth not only measurably supply this defect, but also enrich and meliorate Spirits; for having prepared your Magnet, we shall give you the use of it in sweetning of Spirits.

Take of any sort of ill smelling Spirit or Brandy made from Corn, one part, of pure spring Water two parts, mix them together, that so the stinking and ingrateful Savours may diffuse themselves into the added Water, having so done, you must again free this Brandy thus tempered with the Water, by putting your Magnet thereinto, and so will you draw therefrom all the stinkingness, and 'tis then just as if you had washed that Wine, and rinsed off all its filth, without any charge or difficulty, for the Magnet or exalted Salt desires not to contract friendship with any Impurity.

rity. *N. B.* It remaining the ſame as before, being freed from its Flegm; ſo that this Work is neither chargeable nor difficult; therefore the principal Buſineſs is to be Maſter of ſuch a Salt, the Vertues whereof are known by Experience, becauſe ſome Years ago we have prepared it, and are now again preparing of it, although at preſent the quantity that we have by us is very inconſiderable, as having loſt above two pound three ounces of it by the miſfortunate breaking of a Glaſs, in a conſiderable Tryal, for which great loſs we often lament our unhappy Miſchance; ſeeing we might have been more wary in making ſmaller Tryals, but this we ſhall paſs by, hoping that Providence may in due time multiply our Stores; if not, we muſt learn to be content, ſubmitting our Will to the Divine Pleaſure, who diſtributes of his Riches and Gifts in his own time, and there is no obtaining of it by force, 'tis his own free Gift, ſo that if it is not again beſtowed on us, we may ſay with *Helmont, God Almighty knows for why, he hath given the Goat ſo ſhort a Tail*; peradventure we uſe not the Tallent beſtowed upon us aright, for we are convinced in our Conſcience, that had we applied it the genuin way, it might have been helpful to hundreds that languiſh, *&c.*

We having run through what is neceſſary to be treated of, as to this Part, ſhall

T con-

conclude the ſame; only we think it convenient to add this following and general Head, containing as it were, a Summary of our Labours, being an Anſwer to the Requeſt of a Perſon of Worth, which is as follows.

Worthy Friend,

IN Anſwer to your earneſt Deſire I have given you the Heads of my Books Printed, and thoſe ready for the Preſs; Firſt, you have our *Britannean Magazine*, or Aſſays to Artificial Wines, which (God willing) we intend ſuddenly to Correct and Enlarge with Experimental Additions: Secondly, *Cerevisiarii Comes*, or the Art of Brewing, containing the Grounds thereof, proved and demonſtrated by ſound Philoſophy: Thirdly, *Chymicus Rationalis*, or the Chymical Art rationally ſtated and demonſtrated by a ſhort, but effectual Courſe, containing the Heads of the chief Medicines ſo highly valu'd: Fourthly, This ſaid Treatiſe, which is the *Art of Diſtillation* compleat, to which is added, *Pharmacopœia Spagyrica Nova*, being a Choice Collection of the Specifick Medicines of the Antients. Fifthly, *Spagyrick Philoſophy Aſſerted*, or the true Phyſical Principles demonſtrated by by way of Anſwer to that Learned Dr. *Boylwharf*, in which the Foundation and Preparation of true Specificks are ſo delivered, as eaſily diſtinguiſhable from thoſe pretended to be ſuch by the *Pſeudo-Chymiſts*, a Work highly neceſſary, and as much deſired, and therefore (God willing) as ſoon as may be ſhall ſee the Light: Sixthly, *Speculum Morborum*, in which you may ſee various Opinions concerning the Original of Diſeaſes, and alſo diſcern the true Nature thereof: Seventhly, *Medicina Rationalis*, or the whole Body of Phyſick rationally ſtated upon a new Hypotheſis; containing not only the Original and Definition of Diſeaſes, but alſo their Cure: Eighthly, *Hiſtoria nova de Theſauro Britanniæ interno Celato*, or a new Hiſtory, containing the yet undiſcovered Myſteries of *England*'s Glory and unſpeakable Riches, which may be obtained by the true advancing of its Vegetables and Minerals, by a multiplying and concentring the Univerſal Spirit: Ninthly, *The Magicians Magazine*, or the Wiſe Man's Store-houſe, containing the chief and profitable Heads of all the Voluminous Writings of the Ancient Philoſophers: Tenthly, *Our Ideas of Divine and Natural Things*, being a Philoſophical Diſcourſe of the Macro, and Microcoſmical World; all which ſhall be haſtned with what poſſible ſpeed can be; ſo that I hope in the mean while you will accept of what is done, for that

our

our Resolutions are to improve our Talent according to the Abilities given, and that for the Benefit of such, as prefer Realities, as they are delivered: For we can truly say in what we have done, we have cleared our Conscience toward the Sons of Art, as for my Rewards, I expect it at the Final End, if I persevere in Christian Duties, only to be the Sentence of *Well done thou good and faithful Servant*; *Henceforth is prepared for thee a Crown of Bliss.* Amen.

FINIS.

BOOKS Printed for, and Sold by John Taylor, *at the* Ship *in St.* Paul's *Church-yard.*

1. COllectanea Medica: Or *The Country Physician*, being a choice Collection of Physick, fitted for vulgar Use, containing, First, A Collection of choice Medicaments of all kinds, Galenical and Chymical. Secondly, Historical Observations of Famous Cures. Thirdly, *Philaxa Medicina*, or a Cabinet of Specifick, Select and Practical Chymical Preparations. In Two Parts, Compleat.

2. The Compleat Practice of Men and Women Midwives; or the true manner of Assisting a Woman in Child-bearing. Illustrated with a considerable number of Observations, by *Paul Portal*, Sworn Chirurgeon and Man-midwife in *Paris*, Translated into *English*, adorn'd with many Copper-plates.

2. *Dictionarium, Rusticum & Urbanicum*: Or a Dictionary of all sorts of Country Affairs, Handicraft, Trading, and Merchandizing; Illustrated with Cuts of all sorts of Nets, Traps, Engines, *Octavo*, *Price* 6 *s.*

3. Dr. *Eachard*'s Works; *viz.* The Grounds and Occasions of the Contempt of the Clergy, with Observations on an Answer; with Mr. *Hobb*'s State of Nature consider'd: To which are added five Letters. The 11th Edition Corrected.

4. The Works of the Right Reverend and Learned *Ezekiel Hopkins*, late Lord Bishop of *London-Derry* in *Ireland*, collected into one Volume in Folio.

5. The

5. The Works of *Josephus*, containing the Life of himself, the *Jewish* Antiquities and Wars, *&c.* Illustrated with a new Map of the Holy Land, and divers other Sculptures, Folio.

6. The Proceedings of the House of Commons, 1701.

7. Miscellany Poems, as Satyrs, Epistles, Love Verses, Songs, Sonnets, *&c.* By *William Wicherley*, Esq.

8. *Boyer's French* and *English* Dictionary in *Quarto* and *Octavo.*

9. *Love's* whole Art of Surveying and Measuring of Land, in *Quarto*, *Price* 4 *s.* 6 *d.*

10. *Mercurius Theologicus*, or the Monthly Instructor; briefly Explaining and Applying all the Duties and Doctrines of Christian Religion, that are necessary to be believ'd and practis'd in order to our Salvation. In 12 Parts. By a Divine of the Church of *England.*

11. Bishop *Usher's* Body of Divinity, being the Sum and Substance of the Christian Religion.

12. *Raphson's Analysis Æquationum Universalis e eo spatio Reali seu ente infinito conamen Mathematico Metaphysicum.*

13. Sir *Thomas Pope Blunt's* Essays on several Subjects. The third Edition, with several Additions.

14. Mr. *Wingate's* Arithmetick, the 11th. Edition, with a Supplement of easie Contractions.

Lightning Source UK Ltd.
Milton Keynes UK
UKHW020301100223
416720UK00002B/498